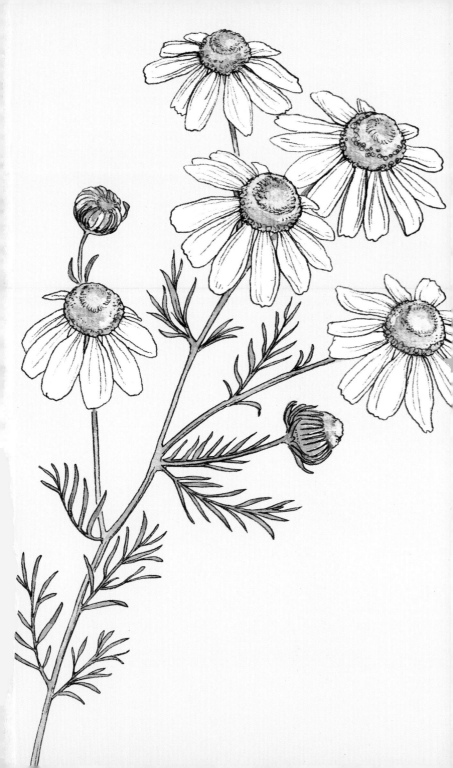

Inspiring | Educating | Creating | Entertaining

Brimming with creative inspiration, how-to projects, and useful information to enrich your everyday life, quarto.com is a favorite destination for those pursuing their interests and passions.

ISBN: 978-0-7603-7791-8
Digital edition published in 2022
eISBN: 978-0-7603-7792-5

The content in this book appeared in the previously published book *The Ultimate Guide to Aromatherapy* (Fair Winds Press 2020) by Amy Galper and Jade Shutes.

Originally found under the following Library of Congress Cataloging-in-Publication Data

Names: Galper, Amy, author. |
Shutes, Jade, author.
Title: The ultimate guide to aromatherapy : an illustrated guide to blending essential oils and crafting remedies for body, mind, and spirit / Amy Galper and Jade Shutes.
Description: Beverly, MA : Fair Winds Press, 2020. | Includes bibliographical references and index. | Summary: "*The Ultimate Guide to Aromatherapy* is a comprehensive guide to using aromatherapy and essential oils for healing written by the co-founders of the New York Institute of Aromatic Studies"—Provided by publisher.
Identifiers: LCCN 2020012697 |
ISBN 9781631598975 (trade paperback) |
ISBN 9781631598982 (ebook)
Subjects: LCSH: Aromatherapy. | Essences and essential oils—Therapeutic use.
Classification: LCC RM666.A68 G35 2020 |
DDC 615.3/219—dc23
LC record available at
https://lccn.loc.gov/2020012697

Design and layout: Laura Shaw Design
Illustration: Abby Diamond /@Finchfight

Printed in China

The information in this book is for educational purposes only. It is not intended to replace the advice of a physician or medical practitioner. Please see your health-care provider before beginning any new health program.

THE
Aromatherapy
COMPANION

A PORTABLE GUIDE TO BLENDING
ESSENTIAL OILS & CRAFTING REMEDIES
FOR BODY, MIND, AND SPIRIT

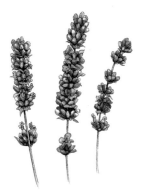

Jade Shutes & Amy Galper
with Amy Anthony, Amandine Peter, and Elisabeth Vlasic

FAIR WINDS

Contents

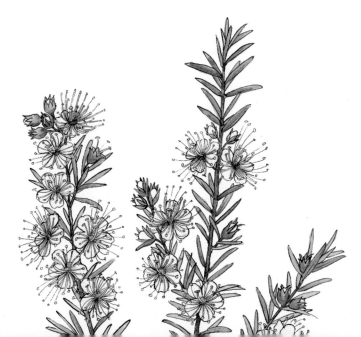

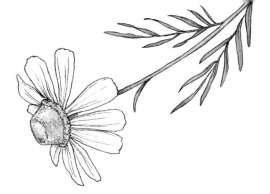

MUSCULOSKELETAL SYSTEM

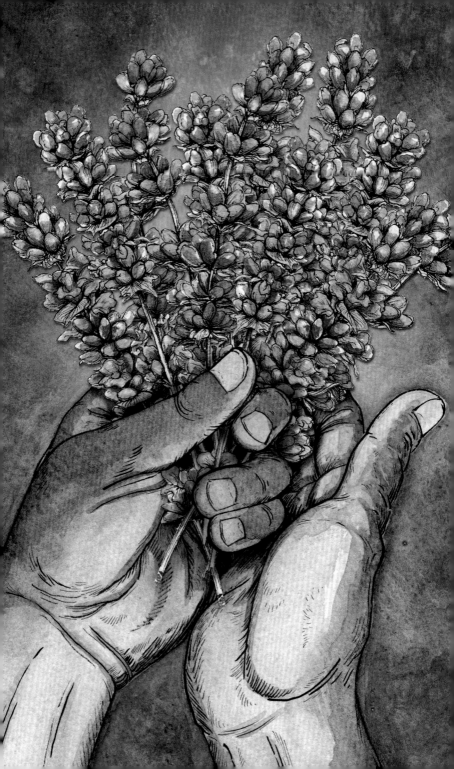

Introduction

EVERYONE IS TALKING about essential oils these days. You can find ample information on them from a variety of media sources that explore their roles in herbal medicine, mindfulness, natural body care, functional medicine, and the practice of Ayurveda and Chinese medicine. But the real challenge is trusting the information you find. Who is writing it? What's their experience?

We've been around a long time, and we have garnered respect from scholars and thought leaders in the field of aromatherapy and beyond. Our students come from around the world. They find us because they want an honest, scholarly, innovative, fun, and balanced approach to learning how to use these remarkable materials.

Our approach is simple: We first celebrate the joy and beauty of the aromas of essential oils. That initial profound connection opens our minds and our hearts to the power (and science) of their medicine. We invite everyone who smells an essential oil to join our mission to connect with our sense of smell and observe how olfaction impacts our well-being and our relationships with plants and with our world.

We love essential oils. This book is our opportunity to share our passion, experience, and knowledge about aromatic plants and their power to impact our lives. Welcome to expanding your journey and deepening your understanding of essential oils!

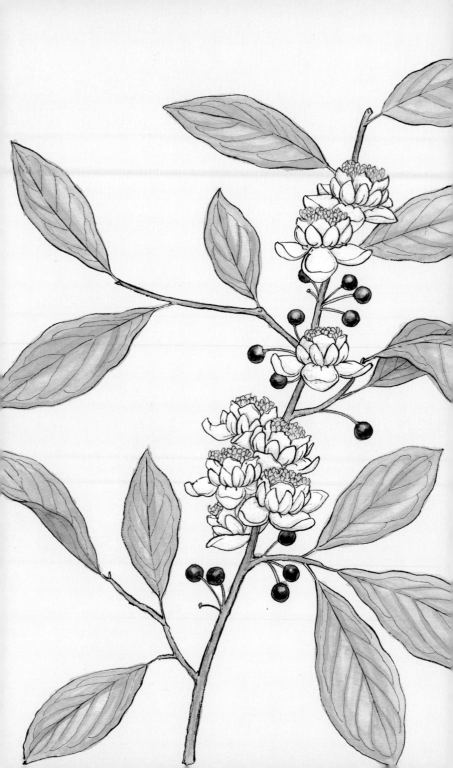

1

Introduction to Essential Oils

WHAT IS AROMATHERAPY? The quick and simple answer—aromatherapy is the study and application of essential oils. It can also be referred to as Essential Oil Therapy, and that's how we like to think of it. Essential Oil Therapy (i.e., aromatherapy) encompasses the holistic application and use of essential oils to support the health and well-being of the individual. We'll use both terms in this book.

Essential oils are highly concentrated aromatic extracts that are distilled or expressed from a variety of plant material, including flowers, flowering tops, fruits/zests, grasses, leaves, needles and twigs, resins, roots, seeds, and woods. They display a set of general physical characteristics that give them their identity:

- Essential oils are highly concentrated, which means they are powerful substances. This is one of the reasons they are diluted into a carrier for application to the skin. Their strength also means a little goes a long way.

- Essential oils are highly complex chemical substances often containing hundreds of unique components. This chemistry is the backbone of the wide range of therapeutic activity essential oils have to offer.

- Essential oils have volatility, which means they can turn from liquid to vapor. Some essential oils, such as citrus oils, are more volatile than others, such as vetiver. This leads us to the next quality.

- Essential oils are light and not greasy. The name essential oil can be deceptive. Essential oils are not vegetable or fatty oils; rather they are light, volatile substances that are referred to as "oils." They have a consistency more like water (although they are insoluble in water) than oil and lack the oily consistency of vegetable oils (except for viscous essential oils, such as sandalwood, vetiver, and myrrh).

- Essential oils are mostly clear to light yellow in color. There are a few blue oils, such as German chamomile, tansy, and yarrow. Patchouli can be dark brown, while inula has a magnificent emerald green color.

WHAT IS THE SHELF LIFE OF AN ESSENTIAL OIL?

- *For monoterpene-rich essential oils* such as citrus oils, conifers (pine, spruce, hemlock), frankincense, lemongrass, neroli, and tea tree: 1 to 2 years

- *For all other essential oils*: 2 to 3 years

- *For viscous essential oils* such as vetiver and patchouli: 4 to 8+ years

ESSENTIAL OIL STORAGE TIPS

- Store essential oils in amber, black, or blue glass bottles to protect them from the potentially damaging effects of light.

- Make sure bottles have an orifice reducer, which helps prevent oxygen from aging the essential oils and helps control the flow of drops.

- Keep essential oils away from light and heat and in a cool place or room to enhance their shelf life and keep their vitality.

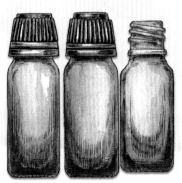

- Essential oils are attracted to and soluble in fatty substances such as vegetable oils (carrier oils), herbal oils, and unscented creams and lotions.

- Some essential oils are thick or viscous. Vetiver is a key example of a viscous essential oil. Unlike a citrus essential oil, which flows out of the bottle, vetiver flows slowly out of the bottle due to its thickness (viscosity). Viscous essential oils are less volatile and tend to have a heavier aroma.

Essential Oil Safety

Our philosophy is that essential oils are safe. It seems simple enough, right? And yet, there are four important caveats:

1. *Essential oils are safe* when selected appropriately for the individual or purpose of the product.

2. *Essential oils are safe* when the appropriate method of application (body oil, steam inhalation, baths, etc.) is chosen for the individual or purpose of the product.

3. *Essential oils are safe* when the correct dilution of the essential oil is used.

4. *Essential oils are safe* when the individual has the appropriate level of knowledge and experience with each essential oil they are using.

Essential oils are powerful. They speak on multiple levels (physiologically and emotionally) to the human organism and are capable of wildly diverse yet complementary therapeutic actions (antispasmodic, anti-inflammatory, etc.). Humans coevolved with aromatic and medicinal plants, which have been our allies as food, as shelter, in magic or ritual, as aromas and olfactory delight, and as medicine. We have a symbiotic relationship. But, like in all relationships, we must cultivate our inherent respect for their power and their potency and use them accordingly.[1]

A POSITIVE APPROACH: ESSENTIAL OIL SAFETY

In his book *Aromatica*, Peter Holmes shares the idea of creating a positive context for essential oil safety. Inspired by his writing, we have adopted and modified his model to create three categories of essential oils for home use as well as for the aromatherapist.

We hope, like Peter Holmes, to inspire a new way of viewing and relating to the safety of essential oils—one through the lens of the *knowledgeable, responsible, reflective,* and *empowered* aromatherapist and essential oil therapist. There are three categories of essential oils:

CATEGORY 1: MILD ESSENTIAL OILS

This category includes most essential oils commonly used at home and in practice. The essential oils in this category are considered to be generally safe and without risk of toxicity or accumulation, even when used over an extended period of time. Specific essential oils in this group may also have unique safety information (e.g., photosensitizer, irritant, etc.).

Mild essential oils

Most essential oils, including cape chamomile, cedarwood, Roman chamomile, German chamomile, citrus oils, cilantro, clary sage, cypress, fir, frankincense, ginger, lavender, lavandin, melissa, pine, rose, saro, tea tree, etc.

CATEGORY 2: STRONG ESSENTIAL OILS

This group of essential oils presents some potential or risk of toxic accumulation of certain components, regardless of method of application. The essential oils below should be used with caution. The main concern is for neurotoxicity (negative impact on the nervous system). Be cautious with dermal applications, be sure to dilute them, and avoid daily long-term application (>10–30 days).

Essential oils in this category are contraindicated (not appropriate for use) during pregnancy or while breastfeeding.

Strong essential oils

- Sage (*Salvia officinalis*), α-thujone, β-thujone and camphor

- Rosemary ct. verbenone (*Rosmarinus officinalis*), verbenone

- Hyssop ct. pinocamphone (*Hyssopus officinalis*), pinocamphone

- Rosemary ct. camphor (*Rosmarinus officinalis*), camphor[2]

CATEGORY 3: POWERFUL ESSENTIAL OILS

Essential oils in this group can cause acute poisoning regardless of route of administration. The oral use of these essential oils should be avoided due to potential for liver and nervous system toxicity. These oils are best avoided unless you have received proper education and training on their use and application.

Powerful essential oils with potential for acute toxicity

- Mugwort (*Artemisia vulgaris*), thujone

- Sage (*Salvia officinalis*), thujone

- *Hyssopus officinalis* NOT *Hyssopus officinalis* var. *decumbens*

- *Lavandula stoechas,* thujone

- Wormwood (*Artemisia absinthium*), thujone

- Cedar leaf (*Thuja occidentalis*), thujone

- Pennyroyal (*Mentha pulegium*), pulegone[3]

Other Safety Issues

Along with the categories above, it is important to also know any specific safety concerns for each individual essential oil you have. And because so many aromatherapy products are applied to the skin, be aware of potential skin reactions. The three main skin reactions are irritation, sensitization, and photosensitization.

> "Ingesting 3 drops of any of these oils constitutes an excessive dose with potentially serious toxicity."
>
> —KURT SCHNAUBELT,
> *The Healing Intelligence of Essential Oils*

IRRITATION

Irritation is when a substance applied to the skin produces an immediate irritating effect. The appearance of the skin may be blotchy and red, and it may be painful or feel like it is burning. The severity of the reaction will depend on the concentration (dilution) and the specific essential oil applied. Avoid using undiluted dermal irritants on the skin, and avoid using even diluted oils on inflamed, open, or damaged skin.

Skin-irritating essential oils include cinnamon bark, citronella, clove bud, lemongrass, oregano, thyme ct. thymol, and winter savory.

SENSITIZATION

Sensitization is either an immediate or, more commonly, a delayed allergic response that involves the immune system. Cinnamon bark (and to some extent, the leaf) and clove bud are good examples of essential oils that can cause both immediate and delayed sensitization responses. Delayed sensitization means that although there may be no reaction upon the first or even after several applications, eventually an inflammatory reaction occurs.

What does it look like on the skin? There will be a red rash or darker area of the skin (in darker color skin), reflecting damage caused by substances such as histamine released in the dermis due to an immune response.[4]

The problem with sensitization is that once it occurs with a specific essential oil, the individual is most likely going to be sensitive to it for many years and perhaps for the remainder of his or her life. The best way to prevent sensitization is to avoid applying known dermal sensitizers to the skin.

Skin sensitizers include cinnamon bark; oxidized oils of pine, fir, and other conifers; and all citrus essential oils.

PHOTOSENSITIZATION

Photosensitization is a reaction to a substance applied to the skin that occurs only in the presence of UV light in the UVA range. Photosensitizing essential oils will cause burning or skin pigmentation changes, such as tanning, upon exposure to sun or similar light (ultraviolet rays). Reactions can range from a mild color change to deep weeping burns. *Do not use or recommend the use of photosensitizing essential oils prior to going into a tanning booth or out into the sun for at least 12 hours after application.*

Certain drugs, such as tetracycline, increase the photosensitivity of the skin, thus increasing the harmful effects of photosensitizing essential oils under the necessary conditions.

Photosensitizing essential oils include angelica root, bergamot, expressed lemon, and expressed bitter orange. Distilled or expressed grapefruit has a low risk for photosensitization.

These citrus oils are not photosensitizing: distilled lemon, mandarin, bergamot FCF, sweet orange, and yuzu (distilled or expressed).

TOP TWO SAFETY TIPS

Know your essential oils! Be sure to have knowledge of each individual essential oil you use.

Recognize the power of dilution! Essential oils are powerful and are often more effective when diluted down than when used undiluted or neat.

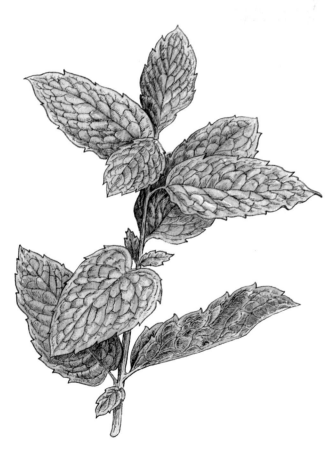

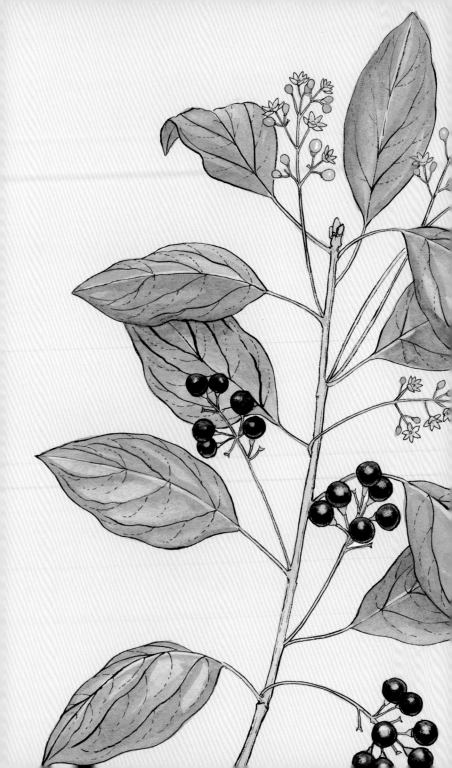

2

The Essential Oils

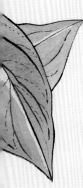

E ssential oils are at the very heart of aromatherapy. These plant-derived aromatics not only support our health and well-being, but they also help us take care of ourselves during times of ill health and emotional stress.

This chapter covers 50 essential oils. Each essential oil mini-monograph contains the following information:

Common name (Latin name, Botanical family): Although they share some common therapeutic benefits, each species of a plant has its own individual chemistry and "personality" and therefore unique therapeutic applications. Knowing the common and Latin name of the plants in each essential oil you purchase is, therefore, important.

Part of Plant: The initial paragraph in each mini-monograph contains the part of plant used in producing the essential oil.

Safety: This section provides safety information relevant to the application of essential oils to the skin, via inhalation, or via diffusion. This section does not contain information relevant to the internal use of essential oils.

Aroma: the aroma of the essential oil

System affinities: the core systems of the body that the essential oil has an affinity with

Blends well with: a list of other essential oils that blend well with the essential oil. This list is a starting point and is not meant to be exhaustive.

Potential substitutions: some ideas on potential substitutions for the essential oil. At times, it may require two essential oils to achieve the same therapeutic activity. We recommend equal drops between the essential oils given. These combinations have been included.

ABOUT SYSTEM AFFINITIES

We believe that each essential oil has very specific affinities to systems of the body. And although each essential oil we cover is capable of affecting a variety of systems, we've chosen to focus on what that essential oil is the best at. Please remember, though, that this is meant as a starting point to get to know the heart of each essential oil and then you can move freely around and beyond.

Therapeutic Applications: This section focuses on the system affinity of the essential oil, along with its psyche/emotional benefits.

- **Indications:** This section highlights indications broken down into different systems of the body. The indications are not meant to be exhaustive. In this section we also include other systems of the body that, although they may not be core system affinities, are still systems we would think about for that specific essential oil, mostly as a support essential oil.

- **Method of application:** These are the recommended methods of application for the system. Please note that the term *personal inhaler* includes an alternative to plastic—smelling salts.

- **Pairs with:** This lists the "Blends well with" essential oils that support and enhance specific systems of the body.

Now, on to the exciting part: getting to know the essential oils! We are about to dive into specific essential oils. Some you may have, some you may be ordering, and some you may hope one day to purchase (e.g., rose essential oil; it's expensive!). We recommend getting any that you do own out while reading about them.

Here's our approach to getting to know an essential oil through our nose, our sense of smell. Begin with the awareness that essential oils are very powerful, and each of us has a different level of sensitivity when it comes to aromas. Hold the open bottle approximately 4 to 5 inches (10 to 13 cm) away from your nose, then move it closer as needed to get the full aroma. As you hold the bottle of essential oil below your nose, gently move it back and forth between your left and right nostrils. This way you will receive the full spectrum of aroma the oil has to give. The aroma should continue to expand as you continue to smell. Pay attention to its several layers. This process only takes a minute or two, but it is the beginning of developing your olfactory palate, so to speak. Now, onwards to the essential oils.

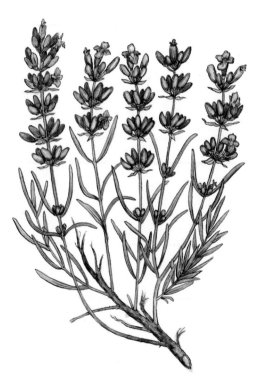

OXIDIZING OILS

Throughout the essential oil mini-monographs, you will come across safety messages regarding when certain essential oils oxidize. What happens when an essential oil oxidizes? And how do you know when it does? There are certain components (e.g., some monoterpenes) that, over time and as they are exposed to air, become oxidized.

Unfortunately, it can be challenging to know when an essential oil oxidizes. Often skin irritation can be the first sign. Other potential signs include a change in the aroma. Just think about how we know when food or carrier oils have gone off. They begin to smell differently—sometimes downright horrible. With essential oils, the aroma may begin to change as it oxidizes, and it may begin to thicken or become more viscous.

For essential oils that have this concern, the dermal safety note will state, "Oxidized citrus essential oils, such as bergamot, should not be used in body care products for application to the skin. The essential oil can, however, be used for cleaning products."

THE SHELF LIFE OF ESSENTIAL OILS

- *For monoterpene-rich essential oils*, e.g., citrus oils, conifers (e.g., hemlock spruce), frankincense, lemongrass, and neroli: 1 to 2 years

- *For all other essential oils*: 2 to 3 years

- *For viscous essential oils*, e.g., vetiver and patchouli: 4 to 8+ years

BLACK PEPPER

Distilled using dried black peppercorns, **Black Pepper** (*Piper nigrum*, Piperaceae) essential oil shines in its ability to support healthy circulation and digestion. Warm and spicy, black pepper essential oil also has pain relieving activity, making it a great addition to muscular aches and pains remedies. The aroma of black pepper seems to be all about will, strength, and empowerment.

DERMAL CAUTION: Potential skin sensitizer if the oil is oxidized. The shelf life is 1 to 2 years. Avoid older oils and store correctly.

AROMA: Pungent, peppery, spicy, warming

SYSTEM AFFINITIES: Circulatory, digestive, musculoskeletal

BLENDS WELL WITH: Clove, Ginger, Grapefruit, Laurel, Lemon, Mandarin, Neroli, Niaouli, Rose, Rosemary ct. cineole or Rosemary ct. camphor, Sweet Marjoram

POTENTIAL SUBSTITUTIONS: Rosemary ct. camphor

THERAPEUTIC APPLICATIONS

CIRCULATORY SYSTEM: Poor circulation, Raynaud's syndrome, sensitivity to cold. **APPLICATION:** Salt scrub, unscented cream or lotion, body oil. **PAIRS WITH:** Ginger, Grapefruit, Lemon, Rose

DIGESTIVE SYSTEM: Indigestion, excess gas, sluggish digestion, lack of appetite. **APPLICATION:** Personal inhaler, salt inhaler, abdominal oil, diffuser. **PAIRS WITH:** Ginger, Grapefruit, Lemon

MUSCULOSKELETAL SYSTEM: Muscular aches and pains, rheumatism, muscle stiffness, arthritic pain. **APPLICATION:** Body oil, gel, aromatic bath, salve. **PAIRS WITH:** Clary Sage, Laurel, Lavender, Lemon, Sweet Marjoram, Rosemary ct. camphor or Rosemary ct. cineole

PSYCHE/EMOTIONS: Mental fatigue, emotional coldness, apathy, low endurance, nervousness, weakness of will, loss of motivation, emotional exhaustion, indecisiveness. **APPLICATION:** Personal inhaler, aromatic bath, diffuser. **PAIRS WITH:** Grapefruit, Juniper Berry, Lemon, Peppermint, Rose, Rosemary ct. cineole

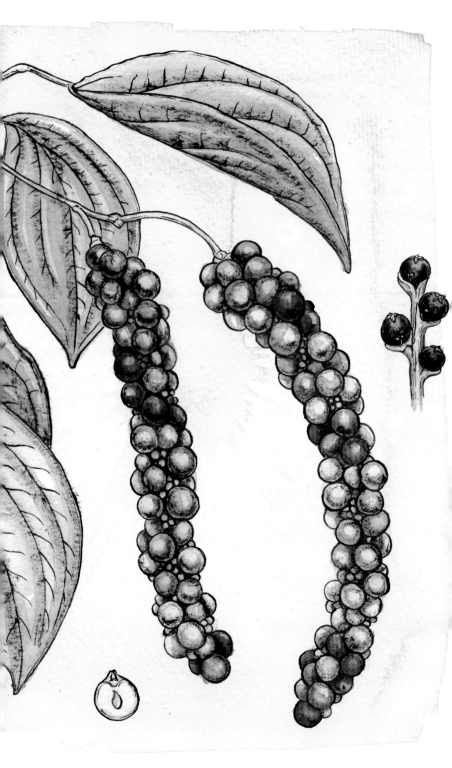

CYPRESS

Cypress (*Cupressus sempervirens*, Cupressaceae) essential oil is extracted from the leaves, twigs, and cones of the cypress tree via steam distillation. Prized for its astringent-like qualities, cypress shines in remedies for varicose veins or skin conditions caused by excess oil (sebum). With its affinity to the respiratory system, cypress can reduce spasmodic coughs and support the body in fighting respiratory infections.

DERMAL CAUTION: Due to the monoterpene content, it is important to store the essential oil properly (in a dark container in the refrigerator or in a cold room away from sunlight and heat). Oxidized essential oils should not be used in body care products or in formulations designed for dermal application. This essential oil can, however, be used for cleaning products.

AROMA: Piney, woody, refreshing

SYSTEM AFFINITIES: Respiratory, circulatory, skin

BLENDS WELL WITH: Bergamot, Black Pepper, Cedarwood, Clary Sage, Juniper Berry, Lavender, Lemon, Sweet Marjoram, Niaouli, Rose, Rosemary, Saro, Black Spruce

POTENTIAL SUBSTITUTIONS: Lemon, Rose

THERAPEUTIC APPLICATIONS

CIRCULATORY SYSTEM: Varicose veins, cellulite. **APPLICATION:** Salt scrub (cellulite), gel (varicose veins). **PAIRS WITH:** Grapefruit, Juniper Berry, Lemon

RESPIRATORY SYSTEM: Coughs, particularly spasmodic dry coughs, bronchitis, asthma, flu, sore throat. **APPLICATION:** Chest salve, undiluted on neck/throat area (sore throats). **PAIRS WITH:** Black Pepper, Cedarwood, Juniper Berry, Lavender, Sweet Marjoram, Niaouli, Rosemary ct. cineole, Saro

SKIN: Oily, sweaty skin and feet, broken capillaries, rosacea, bruises, cellulite, excessive sweating. **APPLICATION:** Facial or body cleanser, gel, unscented cream or lotion. **PAIRS WITH:** Cedarwood, Lemon, Rose

PSYCHE/EMOTIONS: Anxiety, excessive talking, excessive thinking. Deepens yet contracts the breath. Calming, helpful during times of transition and bereavement. **APPLICATION:** Personal inhaler, diffuser, nebulizing diffuser, aromatic baths. **PAIRS WITH:** Bergamot, Black Pepper, Cedarwood, Clary Sage, Lavender, Sweet Marjoram, Rose, Black Spruce

JUNIPER BERRY

Juniper Berry (*Juniperus communis*, Cupressaceae) essential oil is steam distilled using juniper berries and is much prized for its awakening and inspiring aroma.

SAFETY: Due to the monoterpene content, it is important that the essential oil be stored properly (in a dark container in the refrigerator or in a cold room away from sunlight and heat). Oxidized essential oils should not be used in body care products or formulations designed for dermal application. The essential oil can, however, be used for cleaning products.

AROMA: Fresh, piney, fruity

SYSTEM AFFINITIES: Circulatory, musculoskeletal

BLENDS WELL WITH: Clary Sage, Cypress, Himalayan Cedarwood, Blue Gum Eucalyptus, Ginger, Grapefruit, Lavender, Lemon, Lemongrass, Palmarosa, Sweet Marjoram, Rosemary ct. cineole

POTENTIAL SUBSTITUTIONS: Grapefruit, Lemon, Blue Gum Eucalyptus

THERAPEUTIC APPLICATIONS

CIRCULATORY SYSTEM: Poor circulation. **APPLICATION:** Salt scrub. **PAIRS WITH:** Blue Gum Eucalyptus, Ginger, Grapefruit, Lemon, Lemongrass, Rosemary ct. cineole

MUSCULOSKELETAL SYSTEM: Muscular aches and pains, rheumatism, cellulite, joint pain and stiffness, strains and sprains, carpal tunnel syndrome, sciatica, spasms, edema. **APPLICATION:** Body oil, salve, aromatic baths (with sea salts or magnesium salts). **PAIRS WITH:** Clary Sage, Cypress, Himalayan Cedarwood, Ginger, Grapefruit, Lavender, Lemon, Lemongrass, Sweet Marjoram, Rosemary ct. cineole

PSYCHE/EMOTIONS: Fluctuating energy levels, worry, cold, fear, trembling, feelings of being blocked, lack of motivation. **APPLICATION:** Personal inhaler, foot baths. **PAIRS WITH:** Clary Sage, Cypress, Himalayan Cedarwood, Ginger, Grapefruit, Lavender, Lemon, Sweet Marjoram, Rosemary ct. cineole

ROSE

The aromatics of **Rose** (*Rosa × damascene*, Rosaceae) petals can be extracted via hydro-distillation (essential oil), carbon dioxide hypercritical extraction (CO_2 extract), or solvent extraction (absolute). Considered the queen of essential oils, it is often used with emotional imbalances related to menstruation, perimenopause, and menopause. Rose also shines in facial care products. Rose can lift one out of mild depression or help process grief.

SAFETY: No known contraindications or cautions

AROMA: Floral, rich, warm, feminine

SYSTEM AFFINITIES: Female and male reproductive, skin, psyche/emotion

BLENDS WELL WITH: Angelica Root, Bergamot Mint, Black Pepper, Coriander Seed, Celery Seed, Cypress, Grapefruit, Ginger, Himalayan Cedar, Katafray, Lemon, Mandarin, Sweet Marjoram, Neroli, Sweet Orange, Palmarosa, Pink Pepper, Plai, Thyme ct. linalool, Valerian, Ylang Ylang

POTENTIAL SUBSTITUTIONS: Ylang Ylang, Neroli, Jasmine

THERAPEUTIC APPLICATIONS

CIRCULATORY SYSTEM: Varicose veins, broken capillaries. **APPLICATION:** Gel, body oil, cream. **PAIRS WITH:** Cypress, Lemon, Neroli, Palmarosa

REPRODUCTIVE SYSTEM: Irregular/painful menstruation, impotence, sterility, frigidity, reduced/low libido, PMS, amenorrhea, menopause, mild postnatal depression. **APPLICATION:** Personal inhaler, aromatic baths, abdominal oil, body oil. **PAIRS WITH:** Grapefruit, Mandarin, Sweet Marjoram, Neroli, Sweet Orange, Plai, Valerian, Ylang Ylang

SKIN: Broken capillaries, oily skin, mature and sensitive skin, aging skin, wounds, skin blotches, rosacea. **APPLICATION:** Cream, facial oil, gel. **PAIRS WITH:** Cypress, Lemon, Neroli, Palmarosa

PSYCHE/EMOTIONS: Depression, insomnia, shock, anxiety, grief, mood swings, frigidity, lack of libido, heartbreak, anger, frustration, jealousy, resentment, difficulty loving or trusting, lack of creativity. **APPLICATION:** Personal inhaler, roll-on, aromatic bath. **PAIRS WITH:** Angelica Root, Bergamot Mint, Coriander Seed, Celery Seed, Grapefruit, Mandarin, Neroli, Sweet Orange, Pink Pepper, Valerian, Ylang Ylang

VALERIAN

Valerian (*Valeriana officinalis*, Caprifoliaceae) essential oil is steam distilled using the rhizomes (like roots) of valerian. It offers a unique aroma that can lure one to sleep or simply calm and soothe one's spirits after a long day's work.

SAFETY: No known cautions or contraindications

AROMA: Sweet-woody, earthy, sensual

SYSTEM AFFINITIES: Digestive

BLENDS WELL WITH: Angelica Root, Roman Chamomile, Copaiba, Coriander Seed, Cypress, Cistus, Grapefruit, Lavender, Lemon, Mandarin, Sweet Marjoram, Neroli, Pinyon Pine, Vetiver, Ylang Ylang

POTENTIAL SUBSTITUTIONS: Roman Chamomile, Vetiver, Ginger

THERAPEUTIC APPLICATIONS

DIGESTIVE SYSTEM: Nervous indigestion or other digestive issues that arise from stress. **APPLICATION:** Personal inhaler, roll-on. **PAIRS WITH:** Roman Chamomile, Coriander Seed, Grapefruit, Lavender, Lemon

PSYCHE/EMOTIONS: Insomnia, agitation, nervous fatigue, irritability, fatigue. **APPLICATION:** Personal inhaler, roll-on, aromatic bath. **PAIRS WITH:** Angelica Root, Roman Chamomile, Copaiba, Coriander Seed, Cypress, Cistus, Grapefruit, Lavender, Lemon, Mandarin, Sweet Marjoram, Neroli, Pinyon Pine, Vetiver, Ylang Ylang

ANGELICA ROOT

Angelica Root (*Angelica archangelica*, Apiaceae) essential oil is steam distilled using the dried roots of the angelica plant. As a root essential oil, angelica is exceptional for its ability to ground and center one when one is feeling overwhelmed or a bit anxious. Angelica root is the essential oil for supporting and building resilience by keeping one rooted in one's life.

SAFETY: Photosensitizer. The recommended dilution to avoid damage from the sun is approximately one drop of essential oil per 1⅓ teaspoons (6.6 ml) of vegetable or other carrier oil, cream, or gel. We recommend avoiding application to the skin if going into the sun.

AROMA: Sweet, rich herbaceous, earthy, musky, woody

SYSTEM AFFINITIES: Digestive
BLENDS WELL WITH: Bergamot, Black Pepper, Copaiba, Coriander Seed, Fingerroot, Jasmine Absolute, Katafray, Lavender, Lemon, Mandarin, Neroli, Sweet Orange, Patchouli, Petitgrain, Rose, Vetiver, Ylang Ylang

POTENTIAL SUBSTITUTIONS: Lavender + Lemon + Ginger, Celery Seed + Katafray

THERAPEUTIC APPLICATIONS

DIGESTIVE SYSTEM: Indigestion, excess gas, sluggish digestion, lack of appetite, stress-related digestive upsets. **APPLICATION:** Personal inhaler, abdominal oil*. **PAIRS WITH:** Bergamot, Black Pepper, Coriander Seed, Fingerroot, Ginger, Grapefruit, Lavender, Lemon

PSYCHE/EMOTIONS: Nervous tension or upset, irritability, anxiety, insomnia, nervousness, sleep disturbances, emotional ups and downs, feelings of being overwhelmed. **APPLICATION:** Roll-on*, body oil*, personal inhaler, aromatic baths*. **PAIRS WITH:** Bergamot, Coriander Seed, Jasmine Absolute, Katafray, Lavender, Lemon, Mandarin, Neroli, Sweet Orange, Patchouli, Petitgrain, Rose, Vetiver, Ylang Ylang

Refer to safety information above.

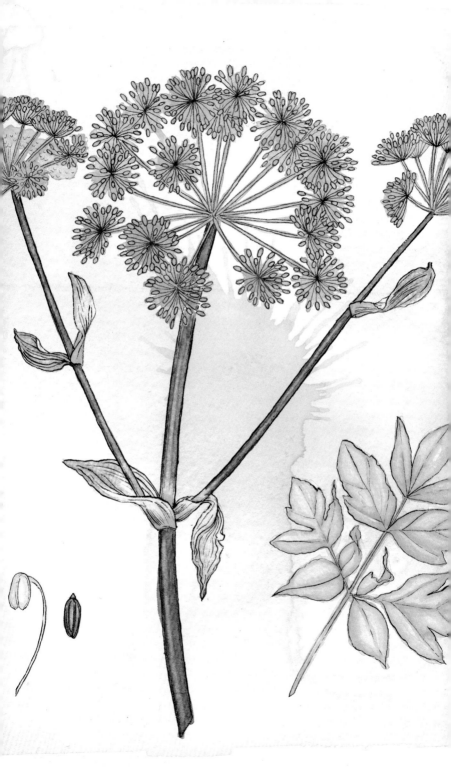

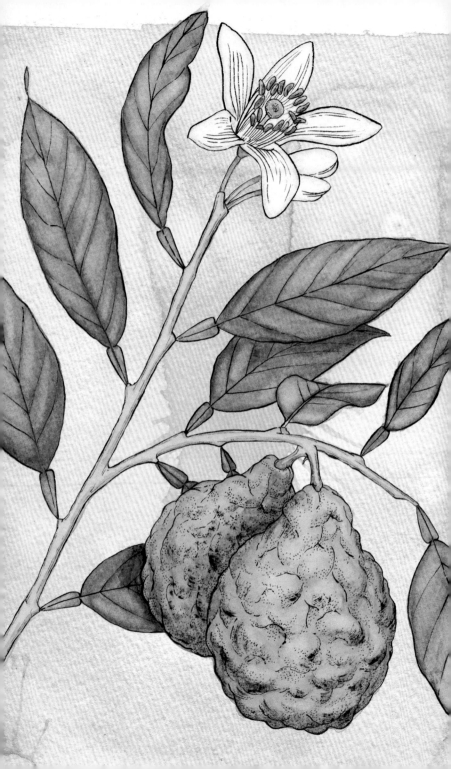

BERGAMOT

Bergamot (*Citrus bergamia*, Rutaceae) essential oil can be distilled or expressed using the zest of the bergamot fruit. The bergamot tree is native to southern Italy, where the best bergamot essential oil is found. Few essential oils shine like bergamot in the realm of emotions. Bergamot calms and soothes during times of stress while also supporting a balanced energy flow to keep you vibrant and motivated. Blending clary sage and bergamot together would tend to be calming, whereas bergamot with eucalyptus would be stimulating.

DERMAL CAUTION: Photosensitizer. The recommended dilution to avoid damage from sun is approximately one drop of essential oil per 1⅓ teaspoons (6.6 ml) of vegetable or other carrier oil, cream, or gel. We recommend avoiding application to the skin if going into the sun.

DERMAL ALERT: Bergamot has a shelf life of 1 to 2 years when stored correctly. Over time, bergamot oxidizes, increasing the chance of dermal sensitization. Oxidized citrus essential oils such as bergamot should not be used in body care products for application to the skin.

AROMA: Rich, exotic, fresh, sweet, sharp, citrus, becoming spicier after a time

SYSTEM AFFINITIES: Digestive

BLENDS WELL WITH: Angelica Root, Bergamot Mint, Cape Chamomile, Clary Sage, Coriander Seed, Frankincense, Jasmine, Lavender, Lemon, Lemongrass, Neroli, Peppermint, Petitgrain, Ylang Ylang

POTENTIAL SUBSTITUTIONS: Lemon + Grapefruit, Lavender + Sweet Orange + Grapefruit (equal parts), Clary Sage + Peppermint + Grapefruit

THERAPEUTIC APPLICATIONS

DIGESTIVE SYSTEM: Digestive upsets triggered or exacerbated by stress. **APPLICATION:** Personal inhaler, abdominal oil*, diffusion. **PAIRS WITH:** Angelica Root, Bergamot Mint, Coriander Seed, Lavender, Lemon

PSYCHE/EMOTIONS: Anxiety, insomnia, emotional instability (mood swings), mild depression. Supports mental clarity, ability to focus, and memory. Reduces irritability. **APPLICATION:** Bath in the evening*, personal inhaler, diffuser, roll-on*. **PAIRS WITH:** Angelica Root, Bergamot Mint, Cape Chamomile, Clary Sage, Coriander Seed, Frankincense, Jasmine, Lavender, Lemon, Lemongrass, Neroli, Peppermint, Petitgrain, Ylang Ylang

Note: Refer to safety info above.

FINGERROOT

Fingerroot (*Boesenbergia rotunda*, Zingiberaceae) essential oil is steam distilled using the bright yellow rhizomes of the fingerroot plant. Fingerroot is a traditional medicine of Malaysia, Thailand, Indonesia, India, and China, where it has been used for its antimicrobial properties, its ability to reduce inflammation, and its effectiveness on a variety of digestive disorders. The fingerroot essential oil offers many similar properties and more. A beautiful oil to work with, it is simultaneously energizing and calming.

SAFETY: No known contraindications or cautions

AROMA: Warming, camphoraceous, slightly floral with a slight citrus note

SYSTEM AFFINITIES: Digestive, respiratory

BLENDS WELL WITH: Angelica Root, Black Pepper, Clary Sage, Copaiba, Frankincense, Ginger, Lavender, Lemon, Lemongrass, Sweet Marjoram, Petitgrain, Hemlock Spruce, Vetiver

POTENTIAL SUBSTITUTIONS: Ginger, Black Pepper

THERAPEUTIC APPLICATIONS

DIGESTIVE SYSTEM: Sluggish digestion, upset stomach, constipation, nausea. **APPLICATION:** Abdominal oil, personal inhaler. **PAIRS WITH:** Angelica Root, Black Pepper, Ginger, Lemon, Lemongrass, Sweet Marjoram, Petitgrain, Hemlock Spruce, Vetiver

RESPIRATORY SYSTEM: Sinus congestion, bronchitis, cold. **APPLICATION:** Steam inhalation. **PAIRS WITH:** Frankincense, Lemon, Sweet Marjoram, Hemlock Spruce

PSYCHE/EMOTIONS: Anxiety, tension, lack of inspiration, lack of focus, foggy thinking, lack of libido, inability to manifest creative dreams. **APPLICATION:** Personal inhaler, diffuser, roll-on. **PAIRS WITH:** Angelica Root, Black Pepper, Clary Sage, Copaiba, Frankincense, Ginger, Lavender, Lemon, Lemongrass, Sweet Marjoram, Petitgrain, Hemlock Spruce, Vetiver

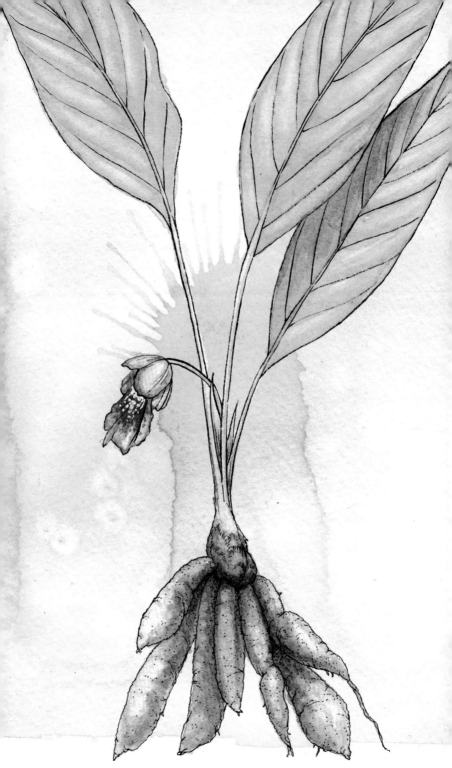

ROMAN CHAMOMILE

Roman Chamomile (*Chamaemelum nobile* syn. *Anthemis nobilis*, Asteraceae) essential oil is a powerful remedy for soothing inflamed conditions of the skin. With its sweet apple-like aroma, it pairs well with mandarin and lavender for a room diffuser or personal inhaler to relax, calm, and encourage a good night's sleep! It is also a powerful remedy for muscle spasms.

DERMAL CAUTION: The likelihood of chamomile preparations causing a contact allergy is low. However, people with known sensitivities to other members of the Asteraceae (Compositae) family (including ragweed, daisies, and chrysanthemums) may want to avoid topical application of chamomile or chamomile products.[6]

AROMA: Sweet, fruity, apple-like, strong

SYSTEM AFFINITIES: Digestive, skin

BLENDS WELL WITH: Angelica Root, Clary Sage, German Chamomile, Katafray, Lavender, Sweet Marjoram, Mandarin, Melissa

POTENTIAL SUBSTITUTIONS: German Chamomile, Cape Chamomile, Lavender, Sweet Marjoram

THERAPEUTIC APPLICATIONS

DIGESTIVE SYSTEM: Stress-related digestive upset or indigestion, bloating, excess gas, stomach cramps. **APPLICATION:** Abdominal oil, personal inhaler, diffuser. **PAIRS WITH:** Angelica Root, German Chamomile, Lavender

SKIN: Inflamed skin conditions, dermatitis, eczema, psoriasis, broken capillaries, acne, slow-healing wounds, razor burn. **APPLICATION:** Facial oil, body oil, unscented cream or lotion, gel, roll-on. **PAIRS WITH:** German Chamomile, Lavender, Sweet Marjoram, Melissa, Thyme ct. linalool

MUSCULOSKELETAL SYSTEM: Spasms, cramps, muscle tension. **APPLICATION:** Body oil, gel, unscented cream or lotion. **PAIRS WITH:** Clary Sage, German Chamomile, Katafray, Lavender, Sweet Marjoram, Mandarin

PSYCHE/EMOTIONS: Anxiety, anger, agitation, stress-related conditions, insomnia, feelings of being overwhelmed, headache or migraine triggered by stress, hyperactivity in children. **APPLICATION:** Personal inhaler, diffuser, nebulizing diffuser, aromatic spritzer, roll-on. **PAIRS WITH:** Angelica Root, Clary Sage, German Chamomile, Katafray, Lavender, Sweet Marjoram, Mandarin, Melissa, Thyme ct. linalool

CORIANDER SEED

Coriander Seed (*Coriandrum sativum*, Apiaceae) essential oil is steam distilled using coriander seeds. Coriander is an annual and herbaceous plant native to southern Europe and western Mediterranean regions. Coriander seed is often associated with digestive upsets triggered or made worse by stress.

SAFETY: No known contraindications or concerns

AROMA: Sweet licorice-like, reminiscent of fennel

SYSTEM AFFINITIES: Digestive, respiratory, nervous

BLENDS WELL WITH: Bergamot, Black Pepper, Cape Chamomile, Roman Chamomile, Ginger, Katafray, Lavender, Sweet Marjoram, Mandarin, Neroli, Sweet Orange, Plai, Palmarosa, Pink Pepper, Rose, Valerian, Vetiver

POTENTIAL SUBSTITUTIONS: Lavender, Bergamot

THERAPEUTIC APPLICATIONS

DIGESTIVE SYSTEM: Indigestion, excess gas, constipation, nausea, stomach cramps, poor appetite particularly when due to stress or feelings of being overwhelmed. **APPLICATION:** Personal inhaler, abdominal oil, roll-on (for stress). **PAIRS WITH:** Black Pepper, Ginger

MUSCULOSKELETAL SYSTEM: General muscular aches and pains, muscular tension from stress or long hours at computer. **APPLICATION:** Body oil, gel, salve, body butter. **PAIRS WITH:** Black Pepper, Roman Chamomile, Ginger, Lavender, Sweet Marjoram, Pink Pepper, Plai, Vetiver

PSYCHE/EMOTIONS: Anxiety, chronic stress, mental fatigue or strain, nervous exhaustion, insomnia, feelings of being overwhelmed, study anxiety, excessive thinking or worry. **APPLICATION:** Personal inhaler, body oil, diffuser, roll-on, nebulizing diffuser, aromatic bath. **PAIRS WITH:** Bergamot, Cape Chamomile, Roman Chamomile, Ginger, Lavender, Sweet Marjoram, Mandarin, Neroli, Sweet Orange, Rose, Valerian, Vetiver

GINGER

Ginger (*Zingiber officinale*, Zingiberaceae) essential oil is steam distilled using dried or fresh ginger rhizome (root). Ginger has a long history of use as a fresh or dried herb and essential oil. It shines in its ability to stimulate digestion, soothe excess gas or bloating, and support timely elimination.

DERMAL CAUTION: No known concerns or contraindications

AROMA: Spicy, warming

SYSTEM AFFINITIES: Digestive, musculoskeletal, respiratory

BLENDS WELL WITH: Angelica Root, Black Pepper, Clary Sage, Clove Bud, Coriander Seed, Jasmine, Grapefruit, Rose, Lemongrass, Sweet Marjoram, Neroli, Plai, Ylang Ylang

POTENTIAL SUBSTITUTIONS: Black Pepper, Spearmint

THERAPEUTIC APPLICATIONS

DIGESTIVE SYSTEM: Stomachache, nausea, vomiting, morning sickness, excess gas, constipation, diarrhea, postoperative or drug-induced nausea, loss of appetite. **APPLICATION:** Abdominal massage oil, personal inhaler, diffuser. **PAIRS WITH:** Angelica Root, Black Pepper, Coriander Seed, Grapefruit, Sweet Marjoram

REPRODUCTIVE SYSTEM: Lack of or reduced sex drive, impotence, menstrual cramps and pain, morning sickness (inhalation), dysmenorrhea. **APPLICATION:** Body oil, personal inhaler, diffuser, abdominal oil. **PAIRS WITH:** Clary Sage, Coriander Seed, Jasmine Absolute, Grapefruit, Rose, Sweet Marjoram, Ylang Ylang

MUSCULOSKELETAL SYSTEM: Muscular aches and pains, arthritis, sprains, rheumatism, joint pain and stiffness, warming. **APPLICATION:** Cream or lotion, body oil, gel, salve. **PAIRS WITH:** Black Pepper, Clary Sage, Clove Bud, Coriander Seed, Grapefruit, Lemongrass, Sweet Marjoram, Plai

PSYCHE/EMOTIONS: Indecisiveness, confusion, frigidity, loss of motivation, burnout caused by chronic stress, lack of direction or focus, feelings of loneliness and resignation, poor memory, foggy thinking. **APPLICATION:** Personal inhaler, body oil, diffuser, unscented cream or lotion. **PAIRS WITH:** Angelica Root, Black Pepper, Clary Sage, Clove Bud, Coriander Seed, Jasmine, Grapefruit, Rose, Lemongrass, Sweet Marjoram, Neroli, Plai, Ylang Ylang

GRAPEFRUIT

Grapefruit (*Citrus × paradise*, Rutaceae) essential oil is expeller pressed or distilled using the zest/rind of the grapefruit and is much beloved for its ability to uplift and inspire. Like all citrus oils, the aroma of grapefruit is used to relieve anxiety while uplifting one's energy and ability to focus.

SAFETY NOTE: Potential skin sensitizer if the oil is oxidized. Avoid older oils and store correctly.

AROMA: Fresh, citrusy, sweet

SYSTEM AFFINITY: Digestive

BLENDS WELL WITH: Bergamot, Bergamot Mint, Black Pepper, Cypress, Blue Gum Eucalyptus, Jasmine Absolute, Juniper Berry, Lavender, Patchouli, Palmarosa, Peppermint, Rosemary ct. cineole, Ylang Ylang

POTENTIAL SUBSTITUTIONS: Lemon, Sweet Orange, Juniper Berry

THERAPEUTIC APPLICATIONS

DIGESTIVE SYSTEM: Constipation, sluggish digestion, digestion-related migraine. **APPLICATION:** Abdominal oil, personal inhaler. **PAIRS WITH:** Black Pepper, Lemon, Peppermint

REPRODUCTIVE SYSTEM: PMS stress and/or tension. **APPLICATION:** Personal inhaler, diffuser, roll-on. **PAIRS WITH:** Grapefruit, Lavender, Lemon, Ylang Ylang

SKIN: Oily/congested skin, cellulite, water retention, hair loss. **APPLICATION:** Cleanser, unscented shampoo, salt scrub. **PAIRS WITH:** Cypress, Patchouli

CIRCULATORY SYSTEM: Sluggish circulation. **APPLICATION:** Salt scrub. **PAIRS WITH:** Blue Gum Eucalyptus, Grapefruit, Juniper Berry

PSYCHE/EMOTIONS: Mild depression, anxiety, stress, nervous exhaustion, agitation, irritability, stress-related conditions. **APPLICATION:** Personal inhaler, body oil, diffuser, roll-on. **PAIRS WITH:** Black Pepper, Jasmine Absolute, Ylang Ylang

SWEET ORANGE

Sweet Orange (*Citrus sinensis*, Rutaceae) essential oil is expressed or distilled using the zest of orange fruit. Sweet orange shines in its ability to uplift and yet calm emotions such as anxiety and stress. Its refreshing aroma also helps to relieve tension or stress-related health imbalances.

DERMAL ALERT: Sweet orange has a shelf life of 1 to 2 years when stored correctly. Over time, the main component of sweet orange (limonene) oxidizes. When this happens, there is an increase in the chance of dermal sensitization. Oxidized citrus essential oils should not be used in body care products for application to the skin. The essential oil can, however, be used for cleaning products.

AROMA: Refreshing, citrusy, orange

SYSTEM AFFINITIES: Digestive

BLENDS WELL WITH: Clary Sage, Roman Chamomile, Himalayan Cedarwood, Coriander Seed, Frankincense, other citrus essential oils, Lavender, Sweet Marjoram, Neroli, Patchouli

POTENTIAL SUBSTITUTIONS: Mandarin, Lemon, Grapefruit, Bergamot

THERAPEUTIC APPLICATIONS

DIGESTIVE SYSTEM: Indigestion, nervous stomach, dyspepsia. **APPLICATION:** Abdominal oil, personal inhaler, diffuser. **PAIRS WITH:** Roman Chamomile, Coriander Seed, Lavender, Lemon, Sweet Marjoram

PSYCHE/EMOTIONS: Insomnia, anxiety, depression, agitation, restlessness, stress, irritability, depression. **APPLICATION:** Personal inhaler, diffuser, nebulizing diffuser, roll-on, aromatic bath. **PAIRS WITH:** Clary Sage, Roman Chamomile, Himalayan Cedarwood, Coriander Seed, Frankincense, other citrus essential oils, Lavender, Sweet Marjoram, Neroli, Patchouli

PEPPERMINT

Peppermint (*Mentha × piperita*, Lamiaceae) essential oil is steam distilled using the leaves. It is stimulating, invigorating, and uplifting. Peppermint essential oil is used to relieve digestive upsets, relieve nausea, reduce muscular aches and pains, and support the respiratory system during the cold and flu season.

CONTRAINDICATION FOR INFANTS: Peppermint essential oil is contraindicated via any route for infants. Avoid application on or near the face of small children due to risk of respiratory spasm and arrest.

AROMA: Fresh, menthol, clean, cool, strong

SYSTEM AFFINITIES: Digestive, respiratory, musculoskeletal

BLENDS WELL WITH: Clary Sage, Coriander Seed, Blue Gum Eucalyptus, Inula, Juniper Berry, Lavender, Laurel, Lemon, Sweet Marjoram

POTENTIAL SUBSTITUTIONS: Juniper Berry, Laurel

THERAPEUTIC APPLICATIONS

DIGESTIVE SYSTEM: Travel sickness, stomach upsets, cramping, gas with abdominal pain, nausea, irritable bowel syndrome. **APPLICATION:** Abdominal oil, personal inhaler. **PAIRS WITH:** Coriander Seed, Lavender, Lemon, Sweet Marjoram

MUSCULOSKELETAL SYSTEM: Muscular stiffness, aches and pains, tight muscles, rheumatism, fibromyalgia, sprains, arthritis, strains, plantar fasciitis, tendonitis, carpal tunnel syndrome, sciatica, bursitis. **APPLICATION:** Body oil, salve, gel. **PAIRS WITH:** Clary Sage, Coriander Seed, Blue Gum Eucalyptus, Juniper Berry, Lavender, Laurel, Lemon, Sweet Marjoram

RESPIRATORY SYSTEM: Bronchitis, sinusitis, spasmodic cough, head cold, common cold, congestion, flu. **APPLICATION:** Personal inhaler, diffuser, nebulizing diffuser, chest salve, steam inhalation (use 1 drop only). **PAIRS WITH:** Blue Gum Eucalyptus, Inula, Laurel, Lemon, Sweet Marjoram, Niaouli, Rosemary ct. cineole or Rosemary ct. camphor, Thyme ct. thymol

PSYCHE/EMOTIONS: Fatigue, foggy thinking/cluttered mind, lethargy, apathy, mental fatigue, difficulty concentrating, tension headache, migraine, travel sickness, shock/trauma, inability to focus. **APPLICATION:** Personal inhaler, roll-on, diffuser. **PAIRS WITH:** Clary Sage, Coriander Seed, Blue Gum Eucalyptus, Juniper Berry, Lavender, Laurel, Lemon, Rosemary ct. cineole

MANDARIN

Mandarin (*Citrus reticulata*, Rutaceae) essential oil is steam distilled or expressed using the peel/zest of the fruit. Mandarin is nurturing and warming, providing a sense of well-being. It's uplifting yet calming.

SAFETY: No known contraindications or cautions. One of the safest oils to use for all ages.

DERMAL ALERT: Mandarin has a shelf life of 1 to 2 years when stored correctly. Over time, the main component of mandarin (limonene) oxidizes. When this happens, there is an increase in the chance of dermal sensitization. Oxidized citrus essential oils should not be used in body care products for application to the skin. The essential oil can, however, be used for cleaning products.

AROMA: Sweet, fresh, citrus

SYSTEM AFFINITIES: Digestive

BLENDS WELL WITH: Black Pepper, Roman Chamomile, Clary Sage, Coriander Seed, Jasmine Absolute, Lavender, Lemon, Neroli, Sweet Orange, Palmarosa, Pink Pepper, Ylang Ylang

POTENTIAL SUBSTITUTIONS: Sweet Orange, Neroli, Lemon

THERAPEUTIC APPLICATIONS

DIGESTIVE SYSTEM: Stress-related digestive upset, dyspepsia, intestinal spasms. May gently stimulate appetite (especially after illness or depression). APPLICATION: Personal inhaler, abdominal oil, diffuser, nebulizing diffuser. PAIRS WITH: Black Pepper, Roman Chamomile, Clary Sage, Coriander Seed, Lavender, Lemon, Sweet Orange, Pink Pepper

REPRODUCTIVE SYSTEM: PMS emotions or stress. Used during labor and delivery to ease tension. APPLICATION: Personal inhaler, diffuser, roll-on, abdominal oil. PAIRS WITH: Roman Chamomile, Clary Sage, Coriander Seed, Lavender, Neroli, Sweet Orange, Ylang Ylang

PSYCHE/EMOTIONS: Tension, insomnia, nervous disorders, mild depression, hyperactivity in children, anxiety, stress, temper tantrums. APPLICATION: Personal inhaler, body oil, diffuser, nebulizing diffuser. PAIRS WITH: Roman Chamomile, Clary Sage, Coriander Seed, Jasmine Absolute, Lavender, Lemon, Neroli, Sweet Orange, Palmarosa, Ylang Ylang

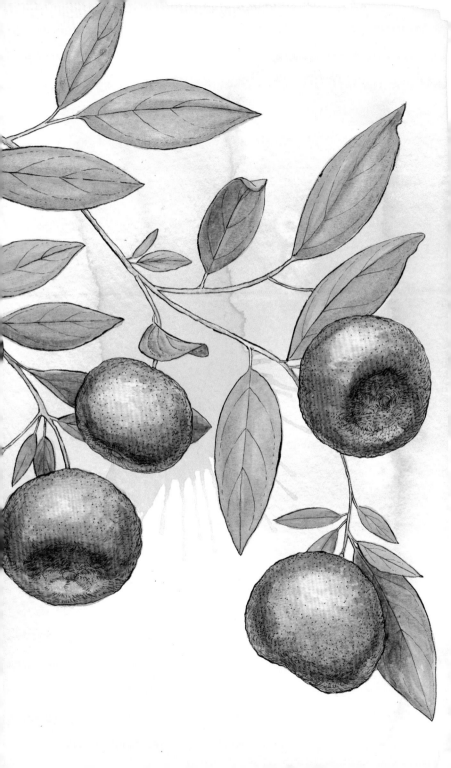

PINK PEPPER

Pink Pepper (*Schinus molle*, Anacardiaceae) essential oil is steam distilled using the dried pink pepper fruits. Although it has "pepper" in its name, it's unrelated to black pepper—though they do share some of the same characteristics. Pink pepper is a relative newcomer to the aromatherapy world. It is used for its pain-relieving activity for sore muscles and general aches and pains. And like black pepper, it supports healthy digestion and promotes circulation.

SAFETY: No known contraindications or cautions

AROMA: Spicy, warming, slightly woody, light citrus

SYSTEM AFFINITIES: Musculoskeletal, digestive

BLENDS WELL WITH: Black Pepper, Roman Chamomile, Clove Bud, Frankincense, Ginger, Jasmine Absolute, Juniper Berry, Lavender, Patchouli, Rose, Vetiver, Ylang Ylang

POTENTIAL SUBSTITUTIONS: Black Pepper

THERAPEUTIC APPLICATIONS

DIGESTIVE SYSTEM: Indigestion, excess gas, sluggish digestion, lack of appetite. **APPLICATION:** Personal inhaler, abdominal oil, diffuser. **PAIRS WITH:** Black Pepper, Roman Chamomile, Ginger

MUSCULOSKELETAL SYSTEM: Muscular aches and pains, rheumatism, muscle stiffness, arthritic pain. **APPLICATION:** Body oil, gel, bath, salve. **PAIRS WITH:** Black Pepper, Roman Chamomile, Clove Bud, Ginger, Juniper Berry, Lavender, Vetiver

CIRCULATORY SYSTEM: Poor circulation, Raynaud's syndrome, sensitivity to cold. **APPLICATION:** Bath, salt scrub, hand or foot cream/lotion, body oil. **PAIRS WITH:** Black Pepper, Ginger, Juniper Berry

PSYCHE/EMOTIONS: Mental fatigue, emotional coldness, apathy, low endurance, nervousness, weakness of will, loss of motivation, emotional exhaustion, indecisiveness. **APPLICATION:** Personal inhaler, aromatic bath, diffuser, roll-on. **PAIRS WITH:** Black Pepper, Roman Chamomile, Frankincense, Ginger, Jasmine Absolute, Lavender, Patchouli, Rose, Vetiver, Ylang Ylang

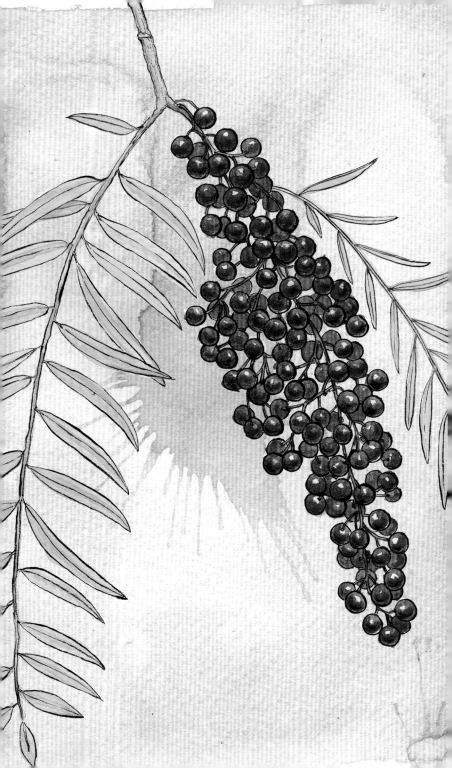

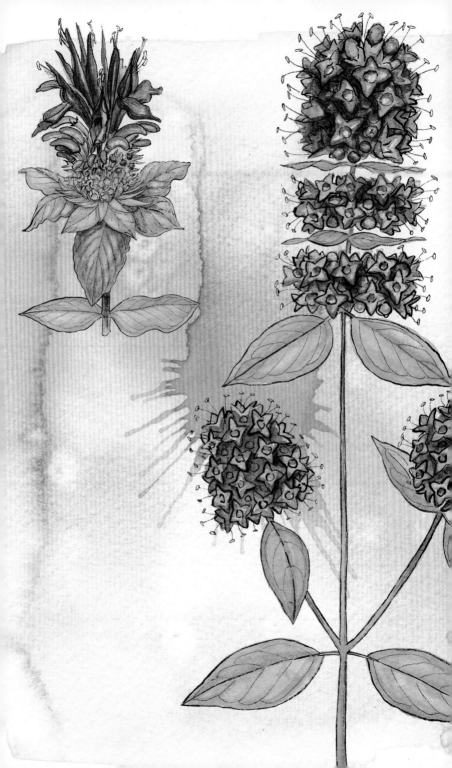

BERGAMOT MINT

Bergamot Mint (*Mentha citrate,* Lamiaceae) essential oil is steam distilled using the leaves of bergamot mint. Reminiscent of lavender with a splash of citrus, bergamot mint essential oil is both energizing and calming. With an affinity to the musculoskeletal system, bergamot mint essential oil can help relieve muscle aches and pains while also reducing tension and the physical or emotional manifestations of stress.

SAFETY: No known contraindications or cautions

AROMA: Soft, lemon-like yet floral, refreshing, slight citrus aroma

SYSTEM AFFINITIES: Muscular

BLENDS WELL WITH: Bergamot, Black Pepper, Roman Chamomile, Clary Sage, Coriander Seed, Jasmine Absolute, Juniper Berry, Lavender, Lemon, Melissa, Sweet Orange, Petitgrain, Pink Pepper, Rose, Hemlock Spruce, Valerian, Ylang Ylang

POTENTIAL SUBSTITUTIONS: Lavender, Clary Sage, Coriander Seed

THERAPEUTIC APPLICATIONS

MUSCULOSKELETAL SYSTEM: Rheumatic pain, muscular aches and pains, muscular tension (e.g., from stress or long hours at the computer), muscular spasms or cramps. **APPLICATION:** Body oil, gel, personal inhaler, unscented cream or lotion. **PAIRS WITH:** Black Pepper, Roman Chamomile, Clary Sage, Coriander Seed, Juniper Berry, Lavender, Lemon, Pink Pepper

PSYCHE/EMOTIONS: Anxiety, chronic stress, mental fatigue or strain, nervous exhaustion, insomnia, stress and stress-related conditions, feelings of being overwhelmed, study anxiety, excessive thinking or worry stress, mental tension. **APPLICATION:** Personal inhaler, aromatic bath, diffuser, aromatic spritzer. **PAIRS WITH:** Bergamot, Black Pepper, Roman Chamomile, Clary Sage, Coriander Seed, Jasmine Absolute, Lavender, Lemon, Melissa, Sweet Orange, Petitgrain, Rose, Valerian, Ylang Ylang

HIMALAYAN CEDARWOOD

Himalayan Cedarwood (*Cedrus deodara,* Pinaceae) essential oil is steam distilled using the wood. Its heavenly earthy wood sweet aroma soothes away tension while calming the mind. Himalayan cedars works well in body care products when a more "masculine" aroma is desired.

SAFETY: No known contraindications or cautions

AROMA: Woody, balsamic, slightly sharp and smoky. Subtle with a hint of spice

SYSTEM AFFINITIES: Skin, musculoskeletal

BLENDS WELL WITH: Bergamot, Bergamot Mint, Black Pepper, Calendula CO_2, Clary Sage, Clove Bud, Cypress, Frankincense, Ginger, Grapefruit, Lavender, Lemon, Lemongrass, Sweet Marjoram, Melissa, Palmarosa, Pinyon Pine, Rose, Vetiver, Ylang Ylang

POTENTIAL SUBSTITUTIONS: Red Cedar

THERAPEUTIC APPLICATIONS

MUSCULOSKELETAL SYSTEM: Muscular aches and pains, muscular tension. **APPLICATION:** Body oil, unscented lotion, gel. **PAIRS WITH:** Bergamot Mint, Black Pepper, Clary Sage, Clove Bud, Ginger, Lavender, Lemon, Lemongrass, Sweet Marjoram, Vetiver

SKIN: Oily skin conditions, acne breakouts. **APPLICATION:** Cleanser, gel, body butter. **PAIRS WITH:** Calendula CO_2, Clary Sage, Cypress, Frankincense, Lavender, Lemon, Lemongrass, Melissa, Palmarosa, Rose

PSYCHE/EMOTIONS: Stress, anxiety, irritability, feelings of being overwhelmed, loss of center. **APPLICATION:** Personal inhaler, aromatic bath, aromatic spritzer, roll-on. **PAIRS WITH:** Bergamot, Bergamot Mint, Clary Sage, Frankincense, Grapefruit, Lavender, Lemon, Sweet Marjoram, Melissa, Pinyon Pine, Rose, Vetiver, Ylang Ylang

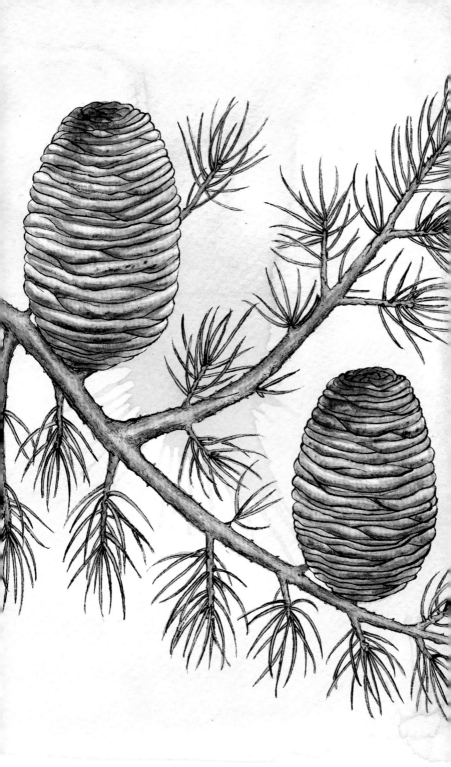

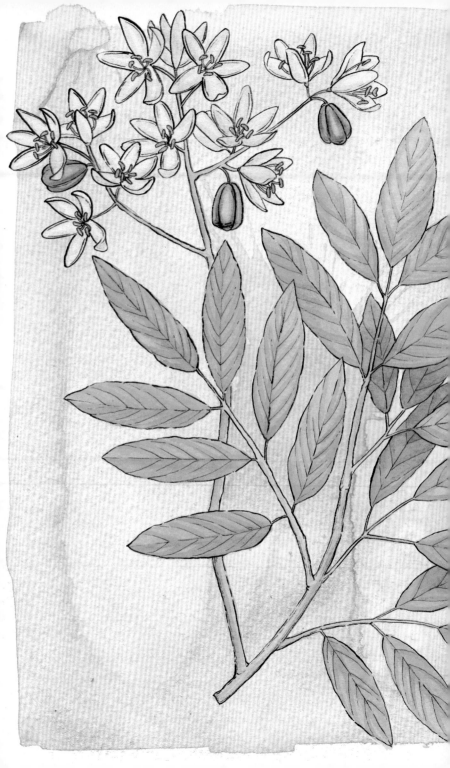

KATAFRAY

Katafray (*Cedrelopsis grevei*, Rutaceae) essential oil is steam distilled using the bark of the katafray tree. Prized for its ability to relieve muscular aches and pains, katafray also soothes and calms tension and irritability.

SAFETY: No known contraindications or cautions

AROMA: Woody with an earthy quality, balsamic, clear and penetrating

SYSTEM AFFINITIES: Musculoskeletal

BLENDS WELL WITH: Angelica Root, Black Pepper, Celery Seed, German Chamomile, Roman Chamomile, Clary Sage, Clove Bud, Frankincense, Grapefruit, Lavender, Lemon, Sweet Orange, Petitgrain, Rose, Valerian

POTENTIAL SUBSTITUTIONS: Lemongrass + Lavender, Black Pepper

THERAPEUTIC APPLICATIONS

MUSCULOSKELETAL SYSTEM: Rheumatism, muscle or joint stiffness, muscular aches and pains, muscle cramps or spasms. **APPLICATION:** Body oil, salve, gel. **PAIRS WITH:** Black Pepper, Roman Chamomile, Clove Bud, Grapefruit, Lavender, Lemon

PSYCHE/EMOTIONS: Nervous tension, irritability, anxiety, nervousness, emotional ups and downs, feelings of being overwhelmed, low self-esteem, lack of focus. **APPLICATION:** Personal inhaler, diffuser, roll-on. **PAIRS WITH:** Angelica Root, Celery Seed, German Chamomile, Roman Chamomile, Clary Sage, Clove Bud, Frankincense, Grapefruit, Lavender, Lemon, Sweet Orange, Rose

PLAI

Plai (*Zingiber cassumunar*, Zingiberaceae) essential oil is steam distilled using the fresh rhizomes of the plai plant. Plai is a newer essential oil to the aromatherapy world, but it makes its mark as an effective pain reliever.

SAFETY: No known contraindications or cautions

AROMA: Earthy, herbaceous

SYSTEM AFFINITIES: Musculoskeletal, respiratory

BLENDS WELL WITH: Angelica Root, Black Pepper, Himalayan Cedarwood, Roman Chamomile, Clary Sage, Copaiba, Coriander Seed, Fingerroot, Ginger, Lemongrass, Sweet Marjoram, Melissa, Niaouli, Sweet Orange, Palmarosa, Petitgrain

POTENTIAL SUBSTITUTIONS: Blue Tansy, Sweet Marjoram

THERAPEUTIC APPLICATIONS

MUSCULOSKELETAL SYSTEM: Rheumatic pain, muscular aches and pains, arthritis, joint pain, cramps or spasms. **APPLICATION:** Body oil, salve, unscented cream or lotion. **PAIRS WITH:** Black Pepper, Himalayan Cedarwood, Roman Chamomile, Clary Sage, Coriander Seed, Ginger, Lemongrass, Sweet Marjoram

RESPIRATORY SYSTEM: Allergies, hay fever, asthma. **APPLICATION:** Personal inhaler, nebulizing diffuser, diffuser. **PAIRS WITH:** Fingerroot, Sweet Marjoram, Niaouli

REPRODUCTIVE SYSTEM: Menstrual cramps, painful menstruation (dysmenorrhea). **APPLICATION:** Abdominal massage. **PAIRS WITH:** Clary Sage, Sweet Marjoram

PSYCHE/EMOTIONS: Stress, anxiety, foggy thinking, confusion. **APPLICATION:** Personal inhaler, roll-on. **PAIRS WITH:** Angelica Root, Himalayan Cedarwood, Roman Chamomile, Clary Sage, Coriander Seed, Sweet Marjoram, Sweet Orange, Palmarosa, Petitgrain

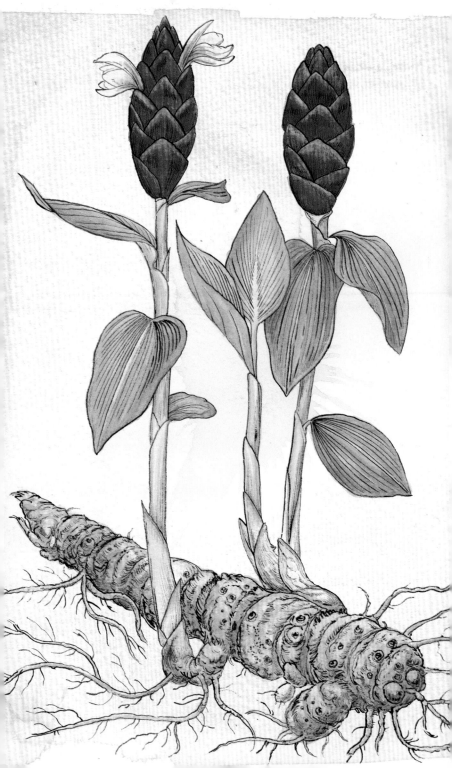

VETIVER

Vetiver (*Chrysopogon zizanioides* syn. *Vetiveria zizanioides*, Poaceae), also known as ruh khus, essential oil is steam distilled using the roots of vetiver grass. Vetiver essential oil can ground one in one's experience and life while relieving the stressors of the day. It provides a sense of focus when one is feeling overwhelmed.

DERMAL CAUTION: No known contraindications

AROMA: Sweet, earthy, warm, woody, deep

SYSTEM AFFINITIES: Psyche/emotion, musculoskeletal

BLENDS WELL WITH: Bergamot, Cistus, Cypress, Fingerroot, Ginger, Grapefruit, Lavender, Lemon, Lemongrass, Neroli, Patchouli, Petitgrain, Pink Pepper, Plai, Rose, Hemlock Spruce, Ylang Ylang

POTENTIAL SUBSTITUTIONS: Patchouli, Ginger, Cypress, Rose

THERAPEUTIC APPLICATIONS

MUSCULOSKELETAL SYSTEM: Muscular aches and pains, sprains, stiffness, muscle tension, arthritis, rheumatism. **APPLICATION:** Body oil, gel, salve, body butter, unscented lotion. **PAIRS WITH:** Ginger, Lavender, Lemon, Lemongrass, Pink Pepper, Plai

CIRCULATORY SYSTEM: Varicose veins, poor circulation. **APPLICATION:** Body oil, salt scrub. **PAIRS WITH:** Cistus, Cypress, Ginger, Grapefruit, Lavender, Lemon, Lemongrass, Pink Pepper, Rose

SKIN: Acne, inflamed conditions, oily skin, irritated skin. Preventative for stretch marks and wrinkles. **APPLICATION:** Facial cleanser, unscented cream or lotion, salt scrub, body butter. **PAIRS WITH:** Cistus, Cypress, Lavender, Lemon, Lemongrass, Neroli, Patchouli, Petitgrain, Rose

PSYCHE/EMOTIONS: Physical and mental burnout, lack of confidence, anxiety, depression. Settles nerves before an ordeal (lecture, dentist). **APPLICATION:** Personal inhaler, aromatic bath, body butter. **PAIRS WITH:** Bergamot, Cistus, Cypress, Fingerroot, Ginger, Grapefruit, Lavender, Lemon, Lemongrass, Neroli, Patchouli, Petitgrain, Pink Pepper, Plai, Rose, Hemlock Spruce, Ylang Ylang

LAUREL

Laurel (*Laurus nobilis*, Lauraceae) essential oil is steam distilled using laurel tree leaves. It inspires and uplifts the spirit and increases focus and concentration. Laurel also has pain-relieving actions for sore muscles/joints and expectorant traits for relieving respiratory congestion.

CAUTION FOR CHILDREN: Avoid application of laurel and other 1,8 cineole-rich essential oils to the face or near the nose of infants and children. Use low dilutions (less than 1%) with children between 3 and 7 years.

DERMAL APPLICATION CAUTION: Use caution when applying laurel essential oil to hypersensitive, diseased, or damaged skin, or on the skin of children under two.

AROMA: Sweet, fresh, slightly minty, camphoraceous

SYSTEM AFFINITIES: Respiratory, musculoskeletal

BLENDS WELL WITH: Bergamot Mint, Cape Chamomile, Cypress, Balsam Fir, Frankincense, Grapefruit, Himalayan Cedar, Inula, Juniper Berry, Lemon, Sweet Marjoram, Green Myrtle, Niaouli, Peppermint, Pinyon Pine, Plai, Rosemary (all chemotypes), Saro, Tea Tree, Vetiver

POTENTIAL SUBSTITUTIONS: Blue Gum Eucalyptus

THERAPEUTIC APPLICATIONS

MUSCULOSKELETAL SYSTEM: Strains, rheumatism, muscle or joint stiffness, muscular aches and pains, fibromyalgia, plantar fasciitis, carpal tunnel syndrome, arthritis, rheumatoid arthritis. **APPLICATION:** Roll-on, body (massage) oil, lotion, aromatic bath. **PAIRS WITH:** Bergamot Mint, Grapefruit, Juniper Berry, Lemon, Sweet Marjoram, Peppermint, Pinyon Pine, Plai, Rosemary (all chemotypes), Saro, Tea Tree, Vetiver

RESPIRATORY SYSTEM: Bronchitis, colds, flu or influenza, viral infections. **APPLICATION:** Steam inhalation, personal inhaler, chest salve, chest oil, aromatic baths. **PAIRS WITH:** Cypress, Balsam Fir, Frankincense, Himalayan Cedar, Inula, Juniper Berry, Lemon, Sweet Marjoram, Green Myrtle, Niaouli, Peppermint, Pinyon Pine, Rosemary ct. cineole, Saro, Tea Tree

PSYCHE/EMOTIONS: Nervous tension, exhaustion, poor concentration or memory recall, depression. **APPLICATION:** Personal inhaler, abdominal oil, diffuser. **PAIRS WITH:** Bergamot Mint, Cape Chamomile, Cypress, Balsam Fir, Frankincense, Grapefruit, Himalayan Cedar, Juniper Berry, Lemon, Sweet Marjoram, Pinyon Pine, Vetiver

LEMONGRASS

West Indian **Lemongrass** (*Cymbopogon flexuosus*, Poaceae) or East Indian Lemongrass (*Cymbopogon citratus*) essential oils are steam distilled using the grass. Chemically very similar, both essential oils are used to relieve muscular aches and pains while also calming stress and relieving tension.

DERMAL CAUTION: Use caution when applying lemongrass essential oil to hypersensitive, diseased, or damaged skin. Always dilute in carrier oil for application to the skin. If you are going to clean with lemongrass in warm water, use gloves!

AROMA: Lemony, strong, herbaceous

SYSTEM AFFINITIES: Musculoskeletal

BLENDS WELL WITH: Bergamot Mint, Black Pepper, Clary Sage, Copaiba, Cypress, Himalayan Cedarwood, Frankincense, Ginger, Jasmine Absolute, Lavender, Palmarosa, Patchouli, Peppermint, Pink Pepper, Plai, Ylang Ylang

POTENTIAL SUBSTITUTIONS: Lemon, Palmarosa

THERAPEUTIC APPLICATIONS

MUSCULOSKELETAL SYSTEM: Muscular aches and pains, tired and sore muscles, sprains, bruises, weakness of connective tissue, pain in joints, muscle weakness. **APPLICATION:** Gel, unscented cream or lotion, salve, body oil. **PAIRS WITH:** Bergamot Mint, Black Pepper, Ginger, Lavender, Peppermint, Pink Pepper, Plai

PSYCHE/EMOTIONS: Fatigue, grieving process, strengthening during weak emotional period, transition, release work. **APPLICATION:** Personal inhaler, salt inhaler. **PAIRS WITH:** Bergamot Mint, Clary Sage, Copaiba, Himalayan Cedar, Frankincense, Ginger, Jasmine Absolute, Lavender, Palmarosa, Patchouli, Ylang Ylang

CLARY SAGE

Clary Sage (*Salvia sclarea*, Lamiaceae) essential oil is steam distilled using the flowering tops of the clary sage plant. Clary sage has a powerful affinity with the feminine and is used for premenstrual tension or mood swings, menstrual cramps, and irregular menstrual cycles. It is also a powerful essential oil for women going through perimenopause, providing strength and a sense of balance. Its pungent floral aroma inspires creativity, acceptance, and joy.

SAFETY: No known contraindications or cautions

AROMA: Sweet, nutty, floral, earthy

SYSTEM AFFINITIES: Reproductive, musculoskeletal

BLENDS WELL WITH: Bergamot, Bergamot Mint, Black Pepper, German Chamomile, Ginger, Grapefruit, Lavender, Mandarin, Sweet Marjoram, Peppermint, Pink Pepper, Plai, Rose, Valerian, Vetiver

POTENTIAL SUBSTITUTIONS: Lavender

THERAPEUTIC APPLICATIONS

REPRODUCTIVE SYSTEM: Menstrual cycle irregularities, PMS and related upsets, cramps, menopause, childbirth/labor, painful menstruation, hot flashes, night sweats, hormonal irritability and imbalance. **APPLICATION:** Abdominal massage oil, personal inhaler, diffuser, baths, hydrosol spray. **PAIRS WITH:** Bergamot, Peppermint, Lavender, Sweet Orange, Ylang Ylang, Petitgrain, Rose, Vetiver

MUSCULOSKELETAL SYSTEM: Aches and pains, arthritis, rheumatism, muscle spasms or cramps, sciatica, carpal tunnel syndrome, plantar fasciitis. **APPLICATION:** Body oil, salve, cream/lotion. **PAIRS WITH:** Bergamot, Peppermint, Lavender, Sweet Orange, Vetiver

PSYCHE/EMOTIONS: Irritability, anger, mental fatigue, anxiety, insomnia, mild depression, mild postnatal depression, exhaustion from overwork. **APPLICATION:** Personal inhaler, abdominal oil, diffuser. **PAIRS WITH:** Bergamot, Bergamot Mint, Black Pepper, German Chamomile, Ginger, Grapefruit, Lavender, Mandarin, Sweet Marjoram, Peppermint, Pink Pepper, Plai, Rose, Valerian, Vetiver

JASMINE ABSOLUTE

Known as the Queen of Night, **Jasmine** (*Jasminum grandiflorum*, Oleaceae) absolute is solvent extracted using jasmine flowers picked at night. The oil is dark orange or brown. This intoxicating absolute not only lifts and inspires the spirits, it is also much admired as an aphrodisiac.

DERMAL CAUTION: Moderate risk of skin sensitization

AROMA: Rich, floral, fruity, heady, exotic

SYSTEM AFFINITIES: Psyche/emotions, reproductive

BLENDS WELL WITH: Angelica Root, Bergamot, Black Pepper, Cypress, Grapefruit, Mandarin, Sweet Orange, Palmarosa, Patchouli, Pink Pepper, Plai, Rose, Ylang Ylang

POTENTIAL SUBSTITUTIONS: Ylang Ylang, Neroli

THERAPEUTIC APPLICATIONS

REPRODUCTIVE SYSTEM: Frigidity and impotence, uterine pain, post-partum depression, PMS, dysmenorrhea (painful menstruation). Facilitates childbirth/delivery. APPLICATION: Personal inhaler, abdominal oil, body oil. PAIRS WITH: Angelica Root, Bergamot, Black Pepper, Cypress, Grapefruit, Mandarin, Sweet Orange, Pink Pepper, Rose, Ylang Ylang

PSYCHE/EMOTIONS: Depression, nervous exhaustion, lack of confidence, lethargy, anxiety, obsessive thinking, tension, agitation, insomnia, loss or lack of libido. APPLICATION: Personal inhaler, roll-on, body oil. PAIRS WITH: Angelica Root, Bergamot, Black Pepper, Cypress, Grapefruit, Mandarin, Sweet Orange, Patchouli, Pink Pepper, Rose, Ylang Ylang

YLANG YLANG

Ylang Ylang (*Cananga odorata*, Annonaceae) essential oil is steam distilled using the flowers of the ylang ylang tree. Ylang ylang is a perennial tropical aromatic tree that originated in the Philippines and has now spread throughout tropical Asia. The essential oil is sometimes referred to as "poor man's jasmine," and indeed it shares many of the same properties and abilities. Ylang ylang is best known for its aphrodisiac qualities, along with being euphoric.

DERMAL CAUTION: Use caution when applying to hypersensitive, diseased, or damaged skin.

CAUTION FOR CHILDREN AND INFANTS: Avoid dermal application of ylang ylang essential oil to children under 2 years of age.

AROMA: Warm, exotic, sweet, heavy, sensual

SYSTEM AFFINITIES: Psyche/emotions

BLENDS WELL WITH: Bergamot, Bergamot Mint, Clary Sage, Frankincense, Ginger, Jasmine Absolute, Lavender, Mandarin, Sweet Orange, Palmarosa, Patchouli, Petitgrain, Rose

POTENTIAL SUBSTITUTIONS: Neroli, Patchouli

THERAPEUTIC APPLICATIONS

REPRODUCTIVE SYSTEM: PMS, low self-esteem, painful menstruation, low libido, PMT (premenstrual tension). **APPLICATION:** Personal inhaler, diffuser, body oil, abdominal oil. **PAIRS WITH:** Clary Sage, Ginger, Jasmine Absolute, Lavender, Mandarin, Sweet Orange, Patchouli, Petitgrain, Rose

PSYCHE/EMOTIONS: Anxiety, anger, bereavement, separation, post-traumatic stress syndrome, nervous tension or depression, frigidity, high blood pressure from stress. An antidepressant; very calming. **APPLICATION:** Personal inhaler, diffuser, roll-on. **PAIRS WITH:** Bergamot, Bergamot Mint, Clary Sage, Frankincense, Ginger, Jasmine Absolute, Lavender, Mandarin, Sweet Orange, Palmarosa, Patchouli, Petitgrain, Rose

BLUE GUM EUCALYPTUS

Indigenous to Australia, **Blue Gum Eucalyptus** (*Eucalyptus globulus*, Myrtaceae) essential oil is steam distilled using leaves and mature branches of the eucalyptus tree. Its strong affinity with the respiratory system makes it the go-to essential oil for respiratory congestion. Eucalyptus is also beneficial for relieving muscular aches and pains and offers an uplifting and energizing aroma.

CAUTION FOR CHILDREN: Avoid application of Blue Gum Eucalyptus and other 1,8 cineole–rich essential oils to the face or near the nose of infants and children under the age of 5 years. Do not instill 1,8 cineole-rich essential oils into the nose of infants or children. Use low dilutions (less than 1 percent) with children aged 3 to 7 years.

AROMA: Strong, camphor-like, balsamic, fresh

SYSTEM AFFINITIES: Respiratory

BLENDS WELL WITH: Laurel, Lavender, Lemon, Green Myrtle, Plai, Peppermint, Rosemary ct. cineole, Hemlock Spruce

POTENTIAL SUBSTITUTIONS: Rosemary ct. cineole, Laurel, Niaouli

THERAPEUTIC APPLICATIONS

RESPIRATORY SYSTEM: Bronchitis, sinusitis, rhinitis, nasal congestion, coughs, cold, flu, pertussis, bronchial mucus congestion. APPLICATION: Steam inhalation, personal inhaler, chest salve, chest oil, aromatic baths.

MUSCULOSKELETAL SYSTEM: Muscular aches and pains, arthritis, rheumatism, plantar fasciitis, sprains. APPLICATION: Gel, body oil, salve. PAIRS WITH: Laurel, Peppermint, Plai, Rosemary ct. cineole.

PSYCHE/EMOTIONS: Foggy thinking, sluggishness, emotional heaviness, lack of energy/vibrancy. APPLICATION: Personal inhaler, roll-on, diffuser, nebulizing diffuser. PAIRS WITH: Laurel, Lemon, Lavender, Peppermint, Rosemary ct. cineole

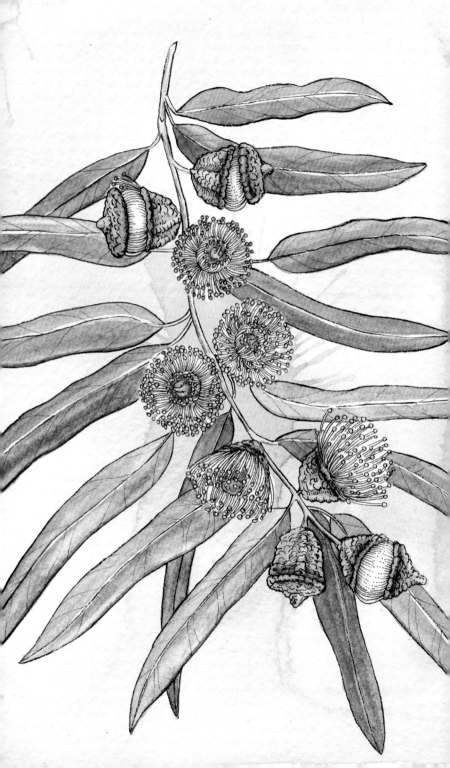

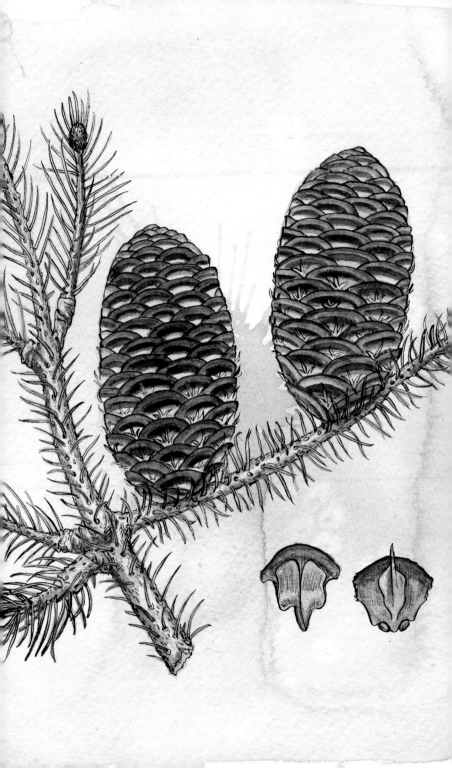

BALSAM FIR

Balsam Fir (*Abies balsamea*, Pinaceae) essential oil is steam distilled using needles and young twigs of the fir tree. This beautiful fir is reminiscent of a forest walk and naturally deepens and expands the breath, reducing stress or anxiety while also gently energizing and uplifting.

DERMAL CAUTION: Potential skin sensitizer if the oil is oxidized. Avoid older oils and store correctly.

AROMA: Fresh, coniferous, pine-like, reminiscent of the forest

SYSTEM AFFINITY: Respiratory

BLENDS WELL WITH: Bergamot, Black Pepper, Blue Gum Eucalyptus, Frankincense, Juniper Berry, Lavender, Lemon, Niaouli, Peppermint, Rosemary ct. cineole or Rosemary ct. camphor, Hemlock Spruce, Tea Tree, Thyme ct. linalool or Thyme ct. thymol

POTENTIAL SUBSTITUTIONS: Other Fir species

THERAPEUTIC APPLICATIONS

RESPIRATORY SYSTEM: Respiratory infections, bronchitis, difficulty breathing, sinusitis, spasmodic coughs. **APPLICATION:** Personal inhaler, diffuser, nebulizing diffuser, chest salve, steam inhalation. **PAIRS WITH:** Blue Gum Eucalyptus, Frankincense, Juniper Berry, Lemon, Niaouli, Peppermint, Rosemary ct. cineole or Rosemary ct. camphor, Hemlock Spruce, Tea Tree, Thyme ct. linalool or Thyme ct. thymol

PSYCHE/EMOTIONS: Mental or emotional fatigue, anxiety. Uplifting, cleansing, clarifying. Relieves stress (by encouraging deep expansive breathing). **APPLICATION:** Personal inhaler, aromatic baths, salt scrub, body oil. **PAIRS WITH:** Bergamot, Black Pepper, Blue Gum Eucalyptus, Frankincense, Juniper Berry, Lavender, Lemon, Peppermint, Rosemary ct. cineole, Hemlock Spruce

INULA

Native to the Mediterranean, **Inula** (*Dittrichia graveolens* syn. *Inula graveolens*, Asteraceae) essential oil is steam distilled using the flowers and flowering tops of inula. This essential oil has a beautiful rich emerald green color. What makes the oil green? When the plant material is distilled in a copper still, some trace components in this oil form complexes with copper, and voilà, the essential oil turns emerald green. When it is distilled in stainless steel, the oil is yellowish clear.[7]

SAFETY: No known cautions or contraindications

AROMA: Fresh, clean, light

SYSTEM AFFINITIES: Respiratory

BLENDS WELL WITH: Blue Gum Eucalyptus, Laurel, Lemon, Green Myrtle, Niaouli

POTENTIAL SUBSTITUTIONS: Blue Gum Eucalyptus, Green Myrtle

THERAPEUTIC APPLICATIONS

RESPIRATORY SYSTEM: Sinus infections, bronchitis, lung congestion, upper respiratory congestion, spasmodic coughs, lethargy, asthma, sinus congestion. **APPLICATION:** Steam inhalation, nebulizing diffuser, personal inhaler. **PAIRS WITH:** Blue Gum Eucalyptus, Laurel, Lemon, Green Myrtle, Niaouli

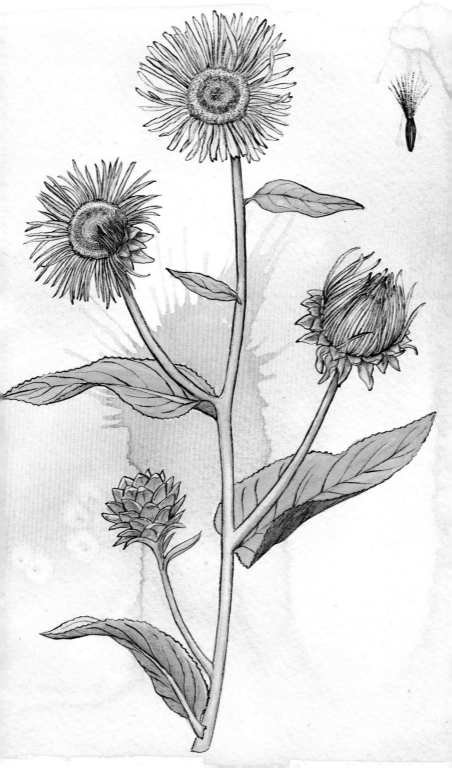

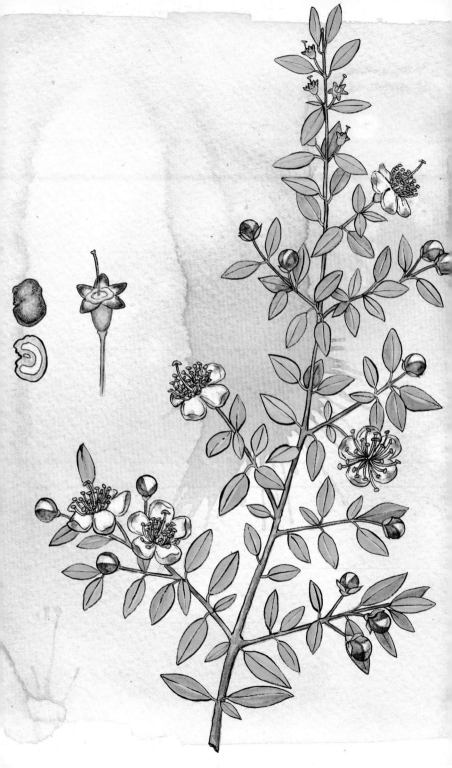

GREEN MYRTLE

Green Myrtle (*Myrtus communis*, Myrtaceae) essential oil is steam distilled using the leaves from the small evergreen shrub. Green myrtle inspires deep and expansive breathing, supports elimination of mucus congestion, and supports the immune system in fighting common respiratory ailments such as the cold or flu.

SAFETY: No known contraindications or cautions

AROMA: Camphoraceous, warm, somewhat sweet, fresh

SYSTEM AFFINITIES: Respiratory

BLENDS WELL WITH: Frankincense, Blue Gum Eucalyptus, Laurel, Niaouli, Rosemary ct. cineole or Rosemary ct. camphor, Saro, Thyme ct. linalool or Thyme ct. thymol

POTENTIAL SUBSTITUTIONS: Blue Gum Eucalyptus, Laurel, Rosemary ct. cineole, Saro

THERAPEUTIC APPLICATIONS

RESPIRATORY SYSTEM: Mucus congestion, bronchitis, excess catarrh, flu, common cold, asthma, chronic smoker's cough, sinusitis, respiratory infections, lung congestion. **APPLICATION:** Steam inhalation, personal inhaler, nebulizing diffuser, chest salve. **PAIRS WITH:** Frankincense, Blue Gum Eucalyptus, Laurel, Niaouli, Rosemary ct. cineole, Saro, Thyme ct. thymol

MUSCULOSKELETAL SYSTEM: Muscular aches and pains, joint stiffness or pain. **APPLICATION:** Body oil, salve, unscented cream or lotion. **PAIRS WITH:** Frankincense, Blue Gum Eucalyptus, Laurel, Niaouli, Rosemary ct. cineole or Rosemary ct. camphor

NIAOULI

Niaouli (*Melaleuca quinquenervia*, Myrtaceae) essential oil is steam distilled using the leaves of the niaouli tree. Popularized by esteemed aromatherapy educator and author Dr. Kurt Schnaubelt, niaouli shines in its ability to support and enhance immunity and the body's ability to deal with infection.

CAUTION: Niaouli and other essential oils high in 1,8 cineole can cause central nervous system and breathing problems in young children. Do not apply to or near the face of infants or children.

AROMA: Camphoraceous, eucalyptus-like with pungent note

SYSTEM AFFINITIES: Respiratory, immune, skin

BLENDS WELL WITH: Cistus, Cypress, Eucalyptus, Lemon, Green Myrtle, Petitgrain, Rosemary (all chemotypes), Saro, Blue Tansy, Tea Tree, Thyme ct. thymol

POTENTIAL SUBSTITUTIONS: Saro, Tea Tree, Laurel

THERAPEUTIC APPLICATIONS

RESPIRATORY SYSTEM: Respiratory infections: bronchitis, colds, sinusitis, chest infections, bacterial or viral catarrhal colds, pharyngitis. APPLICATION: Steam inhalation, personal inhaler, chest salve or oil. PAIRS WITH: Cypress, Eucalyptus, Lemon, Green Myrtle, Rosemary ct. cineole, Saro, Tea Tree, Thyme ct. thymol

SKIN: Acne, athlete's foot, fungal infections, wounds, psoriasis, sores, fissures, boils, scar tissue, ulcers, fungal or parasitic skin infections. Protects from burns from radiation. APPLICATION: Gel, cleanser. PAIRS WITH: Cistus, Cypress, Lemon, Petitgrain, Rosemary ct. verbenone, Blue Tansy, Tea Tree

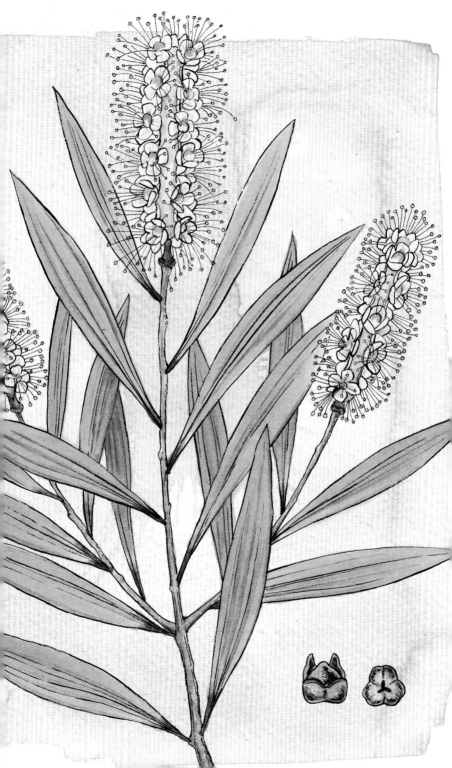

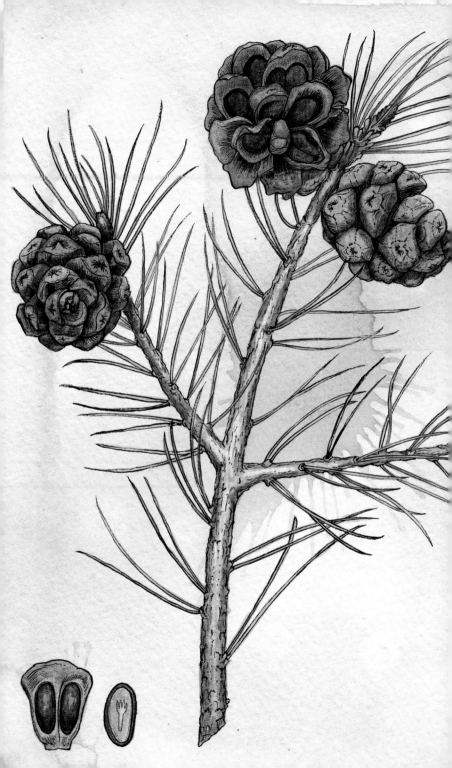

PINYON PINE

Native to southwestern North America, **Pinyon Pine** (*Pinus edulis*, Pinaceae) essential oil is steam distilled using needles, twigs, and branches of this fragrant tree. The resin from the tree can be infused into jojoba oil to make an incredibly aromatic oil that not only relieves muscular aches and pains and respiratory congestion, but also uplifts and inspires!

DERMAL CAUTION: Due to monoterpene content, potential skin sensitization if the essential oil oxidizes. Avoid old or oxidized essential oils.

AROMA: Soft floral-fruity, balsamic, resin-like, earthy

SYSTEM AFFINITIES: Respiratory

BLENDS WELL WITH: Angelica Root, Himalayan Cedarwood, Cistus, Copaiba, Cypress, Balsam Fir, Frankincense, Grapefruit, Lemon, Patchouli, Hemlock Spruce, Saro, Valerian

POTENTIAL SUBSTITUTIONS: Balsam Fir, Himalayan Cedarwood, Hemlock Spruce

THERAPEUTIC APPLICATIONS

RESPIRATORY SYSTEM: Asthma, bronchitis, catarrh, coughs, sinusitis, sore throat, allergies. Expands breathing. **APPLICATION:** Personal inhaler, steam inhalation, chest salve. **PAIRS WITH:** Cypress, Balsam Fir, Frankincense, Lemon, Hemlock Spruce, Saro

MUSCULOSKELETAL SYSTEM: Muscular aches and pains, arthritis, rheumatism, joint pain. **APPLICATION:** Gel, lotion, body oil, salve. **PAIRS WITH:** Himalayan Cedarwood, Grapefruit, Lemon, Hemlock Spruce

PSYCHE/EMOTIONS: Nervous exhaustion, fatigue, depression, mental fatigue. **APPLICATION:** Personal inhaler, diffuser, roll-on. **PAIRS WITH:** Angelica Root, Himalayan Cedarwood, Frankincense, Grapefruit, Lemon, Patchouli, Hemlock Spruce, Saro, Valerian

ROSEMARY

Rosemary (*Rosmarinus officinalis*, Lamiaceae) produces three well-known chemotypes: ct. cineole, ct. camphor, and ct. verbenone. Each chemotype of rosemary has a slightly different aroma and affinity but they are often used interchangeably. The ct. verbenone tends to be the most expensive and is used in regenerative skin care.

ROSEMARY CT. CINEOLE

SAFETY: Avoid application of rosemary ct. cineole and other 1,8 cineole-rich essential oils to the face or near the nose of infants and children under the age of 5 years. Use low dilutions (less than 1 percent) with children aged 3 to 7 years.

AROMA: Eucalyptus-like

SYSTEM AFFINITIES: Respiratory

BLENDS WELL WITH: Cypress, Juniper Berry, Laurel, Lavender, Lemon, Green Myrtle, Plai

POTENTIAL SUBSTITUTIONS: Blue Gum Eucalyptus, Laurel

THERAPEUTIC APPLICATIONS

RESPIRATORY SYSTEM: Sinusitis, mucus, bronchitis, congestion. **APPLICATION:** Steam inhalation, personal inhaler, chest salve, chest oil, aromatic baths. **PAIRS WITH:** Blue Gum Eucalyptus, Laurel

MUSCULOSKELETAL SYSTEM: Muscular aches and pains, stiffness, fatigue. **APPLICATION:** Gel, unscented lotion, body oil, salve. **PAIRS WITH:** Bergamot Mint, Juniper Berry, Lavender, Lemongrass, Peppermint

PSYCHE/EMOTIONS: Poor memory, fatigue, foggy thinking, inability to concentrate. **APPLICATION:** Personal inhaler, diffuser, nebulizing diffuser, roll-on, salt scrub. **PAIRS WITH:** Blue Gum Eucalyptus, Laurel, Lemon, Peppermint

ROSEMARY CT. CAMPHOR

SAFETY: Avoid application of rosemary ct. camphor and other 1,8 cineole-rich essential oils to the face or near the nose of infants and children under the age of 5 years. Use low dilutions (less than 1 percent) with children aged 3 to 7 years.

AROMA: Camphoraceous, eucalyptus-like

SYSTEM AFFINITY: Musculoskeletal

BLENDS WELL WITH: Cypress, Juniper Berry, Laurel, Lavender, Lemon, Green Myrtle, Plai, Peppermint, Rosemary ct. cineole, Hemlock Spruce, Thyme ct. thymol or Thyme ct. linalool

POTENTIAL SUBSTITUTIONS: Rosemary ct. cineole, Laurel

THERAPEUTIC APPLICATIONS

MUSCULOSKELETAL SYSTEM: Muscular aches, cramps, spasms, neuralgic rheumatic pain, arthritic conditions. **APPLICATION:** Body oil, salve, gel, unscented cream or lotion. **PAIRS WITH:** Bergamot Mint, Clary Sage, Juniper Berry, Laurel, Lavender, Peppermint, Plai, Vetiver

PSYCHE/EMOTIONS: Low energy, depression, fatigue, malaise, poor memory, inability to concentrate. **APPLICATION:** Personal inhaler, roll-on. **PAIRS WITH:** Juniper Berry, Laurel, Peppermint. Rosemary ct. cineole

ROSEMARY CT. VERBENONE

SAFETY: Avoid application of rosemary ct. verbenone and other 1,8 cineole–rich essential oils to the face or near the nose of infants and children under the age of 5 years. Use low dilutions (less than 1 percent) with children aged 3 to 7 years.

AROMA: Slightly earthy eucalyptus-like

SYSTEM AFFINITY: Respiratory

BLENDS WELL WITH: Cypress, Juniper Berry, Laurel, Lavender, Lemon, Plai, Rosemary ct. cineole, Hemlock Spruce, Thyme ct. thymol or Thyme ct. linalool

THERAPEUTIC APPLICATIONS

SKIN: Rosacea, acne, seborrhea (oily skin with congestion), varicose veins, wounds. Promotes microcirculation. **APPLICATION:** Facial or body cleanser, unscented cream or lotion, gel, facial or body oil, salve. **PAIRS WITH:** Calendula CO_2, German Chamomile, Lavender, Petitgrain, Thyme ct. linalool, Yarrow

PSYCHE/EMOTIONS: Restores psychological balance, clears mind. **APPLICATION:** Personal inhaler, diffuser, roll-on. **PAIRS WITH:** Rosemary ct. cineole

SARO

Saro (*Cinnamosma fragrans*, Canellaceae) essential oil is steam distilled using the leaves of the saro tree. Saro gained its notoriety for its exceptional benefits for the respiratory system. Diffusing saro into your space during the autumn and winter months could help prevent common seasonal illnesses.

CAUTION FOR CHILDREN: Avoid application of saro and other 1,8 cineole-rich essential oils to the face or near the nose of infants and children under the age of 5 years. Do not instill 1,8 cineole–rich essential oils into the nose of infants or children. Use low dilutions (less than 1 percent) with children between 3 and 7 years.

AROMA: Eucalyptus-like, fresh, clean, green, warm

SYSTEM AFFINITIES: Respiratory

BLENDS WELL WITH: Cypress, Blue Gum Eucalyptus, Balsam Fir, Lavender, Lemon, Green Myrtle, Peppermint, Hemlock Spruce, Thyme ct. thymol or Thyme ct. linalool

POTENTIAL SUBSTITUTIONS: Blue Gum Eucalyptus, Laurel, Rosemary ct. cineole

THERAPEUTIC APPLICATIONS

RESPIRATORY SYSTEM: Acute or chronic bronchitis, moist or dry coughs, the common cold, sinusitis. Protective and preventative to common winter ailments. **APPLICATION:** Personal inhaler, diffuser, nebulizing diffuser, steam inhalation. **PAIRS WITH:** Cypress, Blue Gum Eucalyptus, Balsam Fir, Lavender, Lemon, Green Myrtle, Peppermint, Hemlock Spruce, Tea Tree, Thyme ct. thymol or Thyme ct. linalool

PSYCHE/EMOTIONS: Foggy or cluttered thinking, lack of energy, lethargy. **APPLICATION:** Personal inhaler, roll-on, salt scrub. **PAIRS WITH:** Cypress, Balsam Fir, Lavender, Lemon, Green Myrtle, Hemlock Spruce

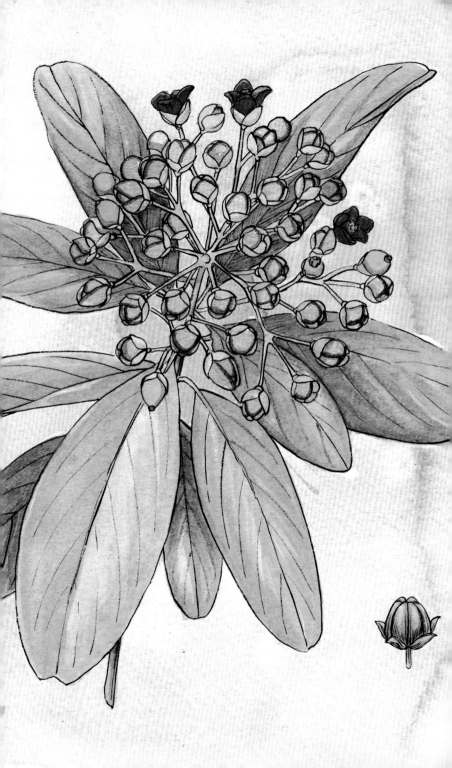

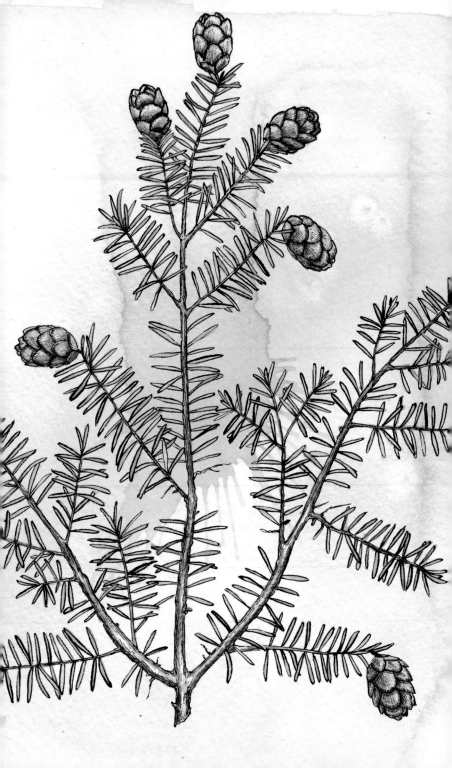

HEMLOCK SPRUCE

Hemlock Spruce (*Tsuga canadensis*, Pinaceae) essential oil is steam distilled using hemlock needles. Hemlock spruce is beneficial when one is feeling burned out and in need of the forest, so to speak. Hemlock inspires deep, expansive breathing while supporting the health of the respiratory system.

DERMAL CAUTION: Potential skin sensitizer if the oil is oxidized. Avoid older oils and store correctly.

AROMA: Pungent, spicy, warming, slightly woody, light

SYSTEM AFFINITIES: Respiratory, musculoskeletal

BLENDS WELL WITH: Balsam Fir, Bergamot, Bergamot Mint, Cistus, Cypress, Fingerroot, Frankincense, Grapefruit, Lemon, Lemongrass, Green Myrtle, Neroli, Pinyon Pine, Rosemary ct. cineole, Saro, Blue Tansy

POTENTIAL SUBSTITUTIONS: Balsam Fir, Pinyon Pine

THERAPEUTIC APPLICATIONS

RESPIRATORY SYSTEM: Colds, flu, bronchitis, catarrh. **APPLICATION:** Steam inhalation, personal inhaler, chest salve, diffuser, nebulizing diffuser. **PAIRS WITH:** Balsam Fir, Cypress, Frankincense, Lemon, Green Myrtle, Pinyon Pine, Saro

MUSCULOSKELETAL SYSTEM: Muscular aches and pains, muscle or joint stiffness, rheumatic pain, tension. **APPLICATION:** Gel, lotion, body oil. **PAIRS WITH:** Bergamot Mint, Grapefruit, Lemon, Lemongrass, Pinyon Pine

PSYCHE/EMOTIONS: Both general and profound fatigue, mental and emotional exhaustion, anxiety, stress. Gives stamina when one is tired. **APPLICATION:** Personal inhaler, roll-on, body butter, salt scrub. **PAIRS WITH:** Balsam Fir, Bergamot, Bergamot Mint, Cistus, Cypress, Fingerroot, Frankincense, Grapefruit, Lemon, Lemongrass, Green Myrtle, Neroli, Pinyon Pine, Rosemary ct. cineole, Saro, Blue Tansy

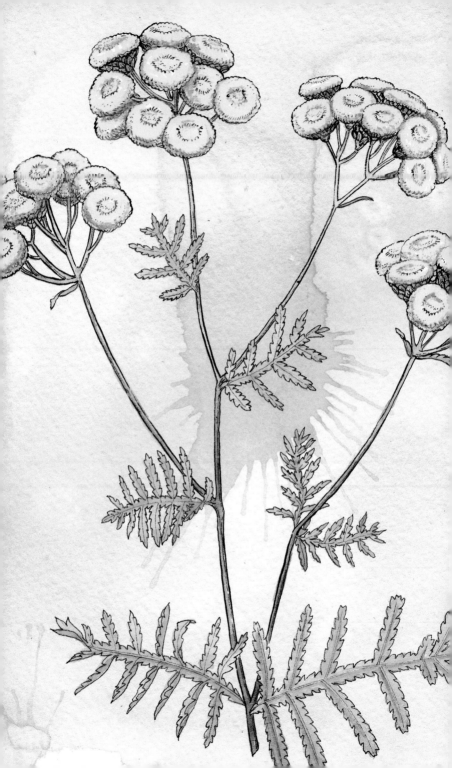

BLUE TANSY

Blue Tansy, also known as Moroccan chamomile (*Tanacetum annuum*, Asteraceae), essential oil is steam distilled using the flowering tops. Blue tansy gained its popularity as an anti-inflammatory, anti-histaminic, and anti-allergenic essential oil used to ease allergy symptoms in the springtime.

SAFETY: No known concerns or contraindications

AROMA: Rich, herbaceous, apple-like sweetness

SYSTEM AFFINITIES: Skin, respiratory

BLENDS WELL WITH: German Chamomile, Coriander Seed, Lavender, Niaouli, Peppermint, Hemlock Spruce

POTENTIAL SUBSTITUTIONS: German Chamomile

THERAPEUTIC APPLICATIONS

RESPIRATORY SYSTEM: Seasonal allergies, hay fever, asthma, emphysema. **APPLICATION:** Personal inhaler, chest salve. **PAIRS WITH:** German Chamomile, Coriander Seed, Lavender, Niaouli, Peppermint, Hemlock Spruce

SKIN: Inflamed skin conditions, itching, itching caused by allergy, eczema, dry irritated skin. **APPLICATION:** Unscented cream or lotion, facial oil, body oil. **PAIRS WITH:** German Chamomile, Lavender, Niaouli

PSYCHE/EMOTIONS: Irritability, easily overheating, anger, frustration. **APPLICATION:** Personal inhaler, roll-on. **PAIRS WITH:** German Chamomile, Coriander Seed, Lavender, Hemlock Spruce

SWEET MARJORAM

Sweet Marjoram (*Origanum majorana*, Lamiaceae) essential oil is steam distilled using the flowering tops of the marjoram plant. Sweet marjoram can help us to accept any deep loss, especially when combined with oils of cypress and rose.

SAFETY: No known contraindications or cautions

AROMA: Spicy, herbaceous

SYSTEM AFFINITIES: Respiratory, musculoskeletal

BLENDS WELL WITH: Angelica Root, Bergamot, German Chamomile, Roman Chamomile, Clary Sage, Copaiba, Cypress, Juniper Berry, Katafray, Lavender, Lemongrass, Mandarin, Melissa, Green Myrtle, Peppermint, Plai, Rose, Rosemary ct. verbenone, Blue Tansy

POTENTIAL SUBSTITUTIONS: Clary Sage, Lavender, Roman Chamomile, Ginger

THERAPEUTIC APPLICATIONS

RESPIRATORY SYSTEM: Spasmodic coughs, bronchitis, sinusitis, flu, allergies, hay fever, colds. **APPLICATION:** Steam inhalation, chest salve, personal inhaler, diffuser. **PAIRS WITH:** Cypress, Juniper Berry, Katafray, Lavender, Green Myrtle, Peppermint, Plai, Rosemary ct. verbenone

MUSCULOSKELETAL SYSTEM: Muscular or joint aches and pains, rheumatic aches and pains, joint swelling, muscle spasms, growing pain (adolescents), cramps, sciatica, carpal tunnel syndrome. **APPLICATION:** Body oil, salve, gel, personal inhaler (to soothe stress). **PAIRS WITH:** Roman Chamomile, Juniper Berry, Katafray, Lavender, Lemongrass, Peppermint, Plai

REPRODUCTIVE SYSTEM: Dysmenorrhea, menstrual cramps. **APPLICATION:** Abdominal oil, personal inhaler, roll-on. **PAIRS WITH:** German Chamomile, Roman Chamomile, Clary Sage, Lavender, Plai, Rose

PSYCHE/EMOTIONS: Anxiety, insomnia, lethargy, nervous exhaustion, stress, agitation/irritability, obsessive thinking, grief. **APPLICATION:** Personal inhaler, aromatic baths, diffuser, nebulizing diffuser. **PAIRS WITH:** Angelica Root, Bergamot, German Chamomile, Roman Chamomile, Clary Sage, Katafray, Lavender, Mandarin, Melissa, Rose

GERMAN CHAMOMILE

This rich blue essential oil is steam distilled using the aromatic flowers of **German Chamomile** (*Matricaria chamomilla* syn. *M. recutita*, Asteraceae). It is beloved for its ability to reduce inflammation, support cellular regeneration and wound healing, and soothe digestive upsets and anxiety.

DERMAL CAUTION: People with known sensitivities to other members of the Asteraceae (Compositae) family (i.e., ragweed and daisies) may want to avoid topical application of chamomile or chamomile products.[5]

SHELF LIFE NOTE: Once it has oxidized, rapidly turning from blue to green and then brown, it should not be used.

AROMA: Sweet, grassy, strong, similar to hay, herby aroma

SYSTEM AFFINITIES: Skin, digestive

BLENDS WELL WITH: Black Pepper, Calendula CO_2, Cape Chamomile, Roman Chamomile, Copaiba, Clary Sage, Lavender, Mandarin, Rose

POTENTIAL SUBSTITUTIONS: Cape/Roman Chamomile, Copaiba, Lavender

THERAPEUTIC APPLICATIONS

SKIN: Eczema or rosacea. Burns. Dry itchy skin, cuts, scrapes, slow-healing wounds, broken capillaries, acne, diaper rash. **APPLICATION:** Cleanser, cream/lotion, gel, salve, facial oil, body oil. **PAIRS WITH:** Calendula CO_2, Copaiba, Lavender, Patchouli, Rose, Vetiver

DIGESTIVE SYSTEM: Digestive upset, cramps, colic pain. **APPLICATION:** Abdominal oil, personal inhaler, roll-on. **PAIRS WITH:** Black Pepper, Roman Chamomile, Lavender, Peppermint

REPRODUCTIVE SYSTEM: PMS, cracked nipples, postpartum anxiety, painful menstruation. **APPLICATION:** Salve, cream, personal inhaler, roll-on. **PAIRS WITH:** Cape Chamomile, Roman Chamomile, Copaiba, Clary Sage, Mandarin, Sweet Marjoram, Rose

MUSCULOSKELETAL SYSTEM: Fibromyalgia, shin splints, spasms or cramps, plantar fasciitis, tendinitis, pain or swelling in joints. **APPLICATION:** Body oil, salve, lotion. **PAIRS WITH:** Black Pepper, Roman Chamomile, Clary Sage, Lavender, Sweet Marjoram, Peppermint, Vetiver

PSYCHE/EMOTIONS: Nervous irritability, mild sleep disorders, tension headaches, agitation/anger, hyperactivity in children; stress-related conditions, anxiety. **APPLICATION:** Personal inhaler. **PAIRS WITH:** Black Pepper, Calendula CO_2, Cape Chamomile, Roman Chamomile, Copaiba, Clary Sage, Lavender, Sweet Marjoram, Patchouli, Peppermint

CAPE CHAMOMILE

Cape Chamomile (*Eriocephalus punctulatus*, Asteraceae) essential oil is steam distilled using the leaves of the cape chamomile shrub. Cape chamomile soothes inflammation, relaxes muscle tension, and relieves anxiety. It has a light blue color due to the presence of a small amount of chamazulene, a component that contributes to its ability to reduce inflammation.

SAFETY: No known contraindications

AROMA: Sweet, fruity, apple-like, strong

SYSTEM AFFINITIES: Skin

BLENDS WELL WITH: Calendula CO_2, Himalayan Cedarwood, German Chamomile, Roman Chamomile, Copaiba, Coriander Seed, Fingerroot, Grapefruit, Katafray, Lavender, Lemon, Mandarin, Neroli, Peppermint, Vetiver, Yarrow, Ylang Ylang

POTENTIAL SUBSTITUTIONS: German Chamomile, Lavender, Roman Chamomile, English Chamomile

THERAPEUTIC APPLICATIONS

SKIN: Itchy or inflamed skin conditions, insect bites, sunburn, acne, psoriasis. May be used undiluted for acute skin conditions such as bug bites, chiggers, and stings, as well as for acne spots. **APPLICATION:** Cream, lotion, body oil for localized application, body butter, gel, salve, roll-on. **PAIRS WITH:** Calendula CO_2, Himalayan Cedarwood, German Chamomile, Roman Chamomile, Copaiba, Lavender, Lemon, Neroli, Yarrow

PSYCHE/EMOTIONS: Anxiety, feelings of being overwhelmed, irritability. **APPLICATION:** Personal inhaler, salt inhaler, diffuser, roll-on. **PAIRS WITH:** Himalayan Cedarwood, German Chamomile, Roman Chamomile, Copaiba, Coriander Seed, Grapefruit, Katafray, Lavender, Lemon, Mandarin, Neroli, Vetiver, Yarrow, Ylang Ylang

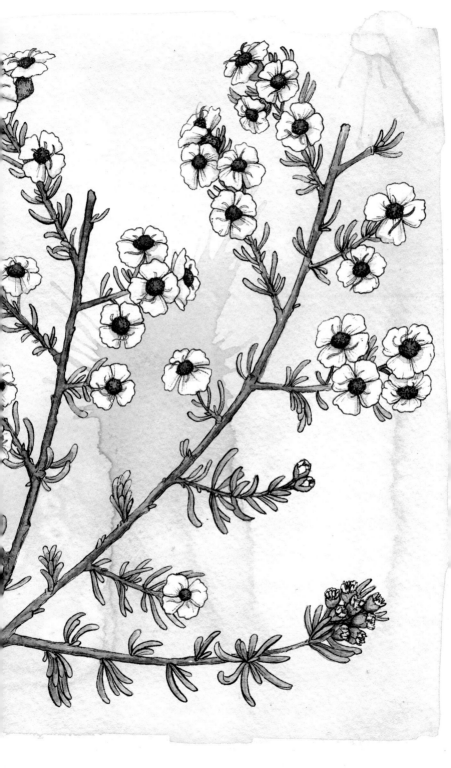

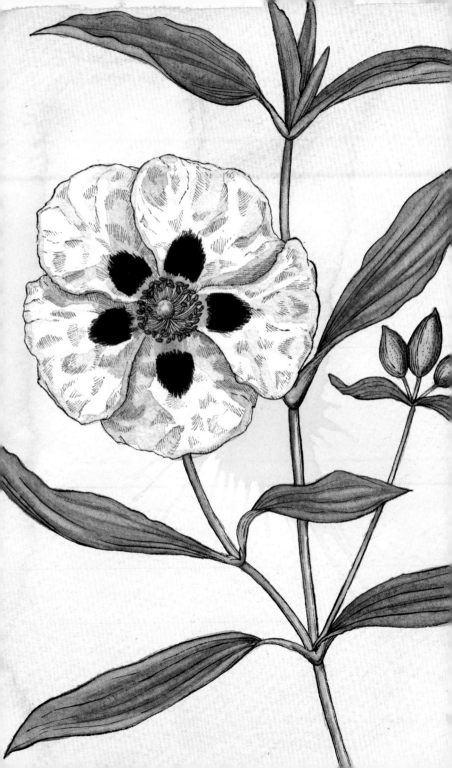

CISTUS

Cistus (*Cistus ladanifer*, Cistaceae) essential oil, also known as rockrose, is steam distilled using the dried delicate cistus flowers and leaves. Cistus essential oil is beloved for its affinity to the skin and wound healing capabilities. Cistus also displays anti-infectious and antimicrobial activity, thereby protecting the wound from infection. We recommend using it in a gel or, if possible, use Cistus hydrosol as a spray for the wound.

DERMAL CAUTION: Potential skin sensitizer if the oil is oxidized. Avoid older oils and store correctly.

AROMA: Warm, woody, herbaceous, crisp

SYSTEM AFFINITIES: Skin

BLENDS WELL WITH: Clary Sage, Frankincense, Katafray, Lavender, Lemon, Neroli, Sweet Orange, Patchouli, Petitgrain, Rose, Rosemary ct. verbenone, Yarrow

POTENTIAL SUBSTITUTIONS: Yarrow, Lavender

THERAPEUTIC APPLICATIONS

SKIN: Cuts, rosacea, broken capillaries, wounds, acne, aging skin, mature skin, prematurely aging skin. **APPLICATION:** Unscented cream or lotion, facial or body oil, gel. **PAIRS WITH:** Frankincense, Lavender, Lemon, Neroli, Patchouli, Rose, Rosemary ct. verbenone, Yarrow

PSYCHE/EMOTIONS: Emotional trauma, old emotional wounds. **APPLICATION:** Personal inhaler, roll-on. **PAIRS WITH:** Frankincense, Katafray, Lavender, Lemon, Neroli, Sweet Orange, Patchouli, Petitgrain, Rose, Yarrow

COPAIBA

Copaiba (*Copaifera officinalis*, Fabaceae) essential oil is steam distilled using the resin that exudes from the cut bark of the copaiba tree. Much loved for its anti-inflammatory activity, copaiba is often used in body care products designed for inflamed conditions of the skin. With its gentle aroma, it also calms and soothes the nerves.

SAFETY: No known contraindications or cautions

AROMA: Resinous, fresh, earthy, heavy, sweet

SYSTEM AFFINITIES: Skin, musculoskeletal

BLENDS WELL WITH: Angelica Root, Calendula CO_2, Cape Chamomile, Cistus, Cypress, Frankincense, Grapefruit, Lavender, Lemon, Lemongrass, Sweet Marjoram, Sweet Orange, Petitgrain, Pinyon Pine, Thyme ct. linalool, Valerian, Yarrow, Ylang Ylang

POTENTIAL SUBSTITUTIONS: Black Pepper, Melissa, Ylang Ylang

THERAPEUTIC APPLICATIONS

SKIN: Mature skin, wrinkles, scar tissue, wounds, eczema, psoriasis, acne, inflamed skin conditions, insect bites. Soothing to dry, irritated skin. **APPLICATION:** Body or facial oil, body butter, aromatic gel, salve, unscented cleanser, cream or lotion. **PAIRS WITH:** Calendula CO_2, Cape Chamomile, Cistus, Cypress, Frankincense, Lavender, Lemon, Lemongrass, Petitgrain, Thyme ct. linalool, Yarrow

PSYCHE/EMOTIONS: Anxiety, tension, inability to focus, irritability, anger, frustration, feeling overwhelmed by stress or pressure. Supports reflection and introspection. **APPLICATION:** Personal inhaler, roll-on, aromatic spritzer. **PAIRS WITH:** Angelica Root, Cape Chamomile, Cistus, Frankincense, Grapefruit, Lavender, Lemon, Sweet Marjoram, Sweet Orange, Petitgrain, Pinyon Pine, Valerian, Yarrow, Ylang Ylang

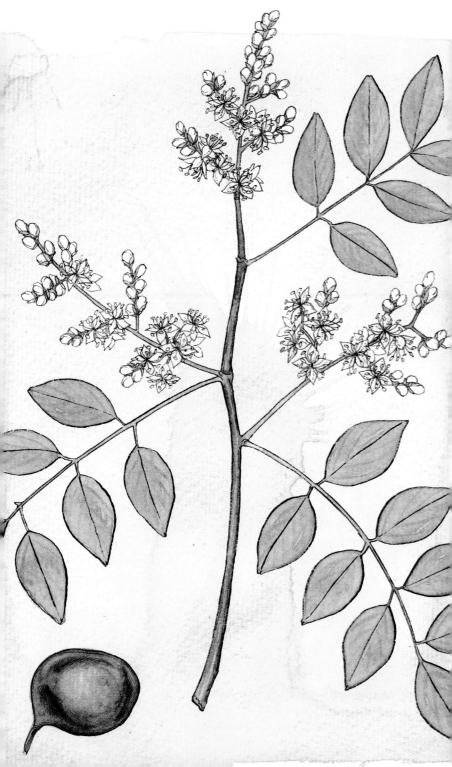

FRANKINCENSE

Frankincense (*Boswellia sacra* syn. *Boswellia carteri*, Burseraceae) essential oil is steam distilled using the resin of the frankincense tree.

DERMAL CAUTION: Potential skin sensitizer if the oil is oxidized. Avoid older oils and store correctly.

AROMA: Clean, fresh, earthy, woody

SYSTEM AFFINITIES: Skin

BLENDS WELL WITH: Bergamot Mint, Black Pepper, Calendula CO_2, Himalayan Cedarwood, Roman Chamomile, Cistus, Copaiba, Cypress, Blue Gum Eucalyptus, Inula, Lavender, Lemon, Lemongrass, Mandarin, Melissa, Neroli, Niaouli, Sweet Orange, Patchouli, Pinyon Pine, Rose, Hemlock Spruce

POTENTIAL SUBSTITUTIONS: Lavender, Cistus

THERAPEUTIC APPLICATIONS

SKIN: Mature skin, wrinkles, scar tissue, postoperative wound healing (once sutures are removed), eczema, acne, inflamed skin conditions, blackheads, hives. Soothing to dry, irritated skin. **APPLICATION:** Unscented cream or lotion, salve, body butter, body or facial oil. **PAIRS WITH:** Himalayan Cedarwood, Roman Chamomile, Cistus, Copaiba, Cypress, Lavender, Lemongrass, Melissa, Neroli, Niaouli, Patchouli, Rose

RESPIRATORY SYSTEM: Bronchitis, sinus congestion, asthma. **APPLICATION:** Steam inhalation, personal inhaler, chest salve, nebulizing diffuser. **PAIRS WITH:** Cypress, Blue Gum Eucalyptus, Inula, Lemon, Niaouli, Pinyon Pine, Hemlock Spruce

PSYCHE/EMOTIONS: Anxiety, tension, inability to focus. Meditative, supports reflection and introspection, healing on all levels of spirit and emotion, stills the mind, promotes spiritual consciousness and tranquility, soothes the spirit. A wonderful oil to demonstrate the mind-body connection. **APPLICATION:** Personal inhaler, diffuser, nebulizing diffuser, roll-on, aromatic bath. **PAIRS WITH:** Bergamot Mint, Himalayan Cedarwood, Roman Chamomile, Lavender, Lemon, Mandarin, Melissa, Neroli, Sweet Orange, Patchouli, Pinyon Pine, Rose, Hemlock Spruce

LAVENDER

Considered the "mother of all essential oils," **Lavender** essential oil is steam distilled using the flowering tops and leaves of the lavender plant, *Lavandula angustifolia* (Lamiaceae). It not only provides a wide spectrum of possible uses, it is considered an enhancer for just about all other essential oils.

DERMAL CAUTION: No known cautions

AROMA: Fresh, floral, sweet, herbaceous

SYSTEM AFFINITIES: Skin, all systems

BLENDS WELL WITH: Most essential oils

POTENTIAL SUBSTITUTIONS: Lavender has such a wide range of activity that is unique to it that it would be challenging to replace. We recommend choosing a substitution based upon what you are looking for the oil to do in the blend/formulation.

THERAPEUTIC APPLICATIONS

SKIN: Burns, scrapes, acne, athlete's foot, eczema, inflamed skin conditions, psoriasis, sunburn, itchy skin, insect bites. APPLICATION: Gel, unscented cream or lotion, body or facial oil, foot bath, lip balm. PAIRS WITH: See System Affinity Review on page 152.

REPRODUCTIVE SYSTEM: Can help reduce severity of labor contractions (use with Clary Sage); helps in relieving menstrual cramps. APPLICATION: Personal inhaler, diffuser, nebulizing diffuser, aromatic bath, roll-on. PAIRS WITH: Clary Sage, Jasmine Absolute, Lavender, Mandarin, Sweet Marjoram, Neroli, Petitgrain, Rose

MUSCULOSKELETAL SYSTEM: Muscular aches and pains, arthritis, sprains, strains, growing pains, plantar fasciitis, tendonitis, shin splints, rheumatic conditions, joint pain and stiffness, bursitis. APPLICATION: Body oil, salve, gel, roll-on, aromatic bath. PAIRS WITH: Bergamot Mint, Black Pepper, Clove Bud, Ginger, Juniper Berry, Laurel, Sweet Marjoram, Peppermint, Rosemary ct. camphor or Rosemary ct. cineole

PSYCHE/EMOTIONS: Irritability, mild depression, anxiety, hyperactivity, panic attacks, insomnia. APPLICATION: Aromatic bath, personal inhaler, roll-on, diffuser, nebulizing diffuser, aromatic spritzer. PAIRS WITH: Bergamot, German Chamomile, Roman Chamomile, Grapefruit, Lemon, Mandarin, Neroli, Sweet Orange, Petitgrain, Pinyon Pine, Rose, Ylang Ylang

LEMON

MUSCULOSKELETAL SYSTEM

Lemon (*Citrus limon*, Rutaceae) essential oil is expressed or steam distilled using the peel or zest. It can be used for uplifting emotions, reducing stress, aiding the body as it fights infection, and supporting overall health.

DERMAL ALERT: Oxidized citrus essential oils such as lemon should not be used in body care products for the skin.

DERMAL CAUTION: Expressed lemon has a very low risk of being photosensitizing; distilled lemon is not phototoxic. Dilution rate for skin products is 12 to 18 drops per ounce of carrier oil or base product.

AROMA: Sharp, citrus, refreshing

SYSTEM AFFINITIES: Digestive, circulatory

BLENDS WELL WITH: Celery Seed, Clary Sage, Cypress, Blue Gum Eucalyptus, Douglas Fir, Fingerroot, Frankincense, Ginger, Grapefruit, Juniper Berry, Katafray, Lavender, Lemongrass, Neroli, Niaouli, Palmarosa, Pink Pepper, Pinyon Pine, Rosemary ct. cineole or Rosemary ct. camphor, Hemlock Spruce, Tea Tree

POTENTIAL SUBSTITUTIONS: Grapefruit, Sweet Orange

THERAPEUTIC APPLICATIONS

SKIN: Acne, premature aging skin (preventative), oily complexions, mouth ulcers, cellulite, rosacea, broken capillaries. **APPLICATION:** Unscented cream or lotion, gel, body or facial oil. **PAIRS WITH:** Celery Seed, Cypress, Frankincense, Lavender, Lemongrass, Neroli, Niaouli, Palmarosa, Tea Tree

CIRCULATORY SYSTEM: Poor circulation, capillary fragility, varicose veins. **APPLICATION:** Salt scrub*. **PAIRS WITH:** Celery Seed, Cypress, Grapefruit, Juniper Berry, Lemongrass, Rosemary ct. cineole

MUSCULOSKELETAL SYSTEM: Muscular or joint aches and pains, arthritis, cellulite, rheumatism, joint swelling, gout. **APPLICATION:** Body oil, gel, salt scrub. **PAIRS WITH:** Clary Sage, Ginger, Grapefruit, Juniper Berry, Katafray, Lavender, Lemongrass, Pinyon Pine, Rosemary ct. cineole or Rosemary ct. camphor, Hemlock Spruce

PSYCHE/EMOTIONS: Anxiety, depression, stress, anger/irritability. **APPLICATION:** Personal inhaler, diffuser, nebulizing diffuser, salt inhaler. **PAIRS WITH:** Clary Sage, Douglas Fir, Frankincense, Grapefruit, Lavender, Neroli, Pinyon Pine, Hemlock Spruce

Do not use on varicose veins.

NEROLI

Neroli (*Citrus aurantium* var. *amara*, Rutaceae) essential oil is steam distilled using the flowers of the bitter orange tree. It was named after the princess of Nerola in Italy, who used the perfumed oil to scent her gloves and bathwater.

SAFETY: No known contraindications

AROMA: Sweet, floral

SYSTEM AFFINITIES: Skin, psyche/emotions

BLENDS WELL WITH: Angelica Root, Bergamot Mint, Calendula CO_2, Celery Seed, Cistus, Copaiba, Clary Sage, Coriander Seed, Cypress, Fingerroot, Grapefruit, Lavender, Lemongrass, Mandarin, Sweet Orange, Palmarosa, Petitgrain, Pinyon Pine, Hemlock Spruce, Valerian, Ylang Ylang

POTENTIAL SUBSTITUTIONS: Jasmine, Petitgrain, Ylang Ylang

THERAPEUTIC APPLICATIONS

SKIN: Oily skin conditions, spider veins, stretch marks, wounds. APPLICATION: Facial oil, cream, lotion, body butter. PAIRS WITH: Calendula CO_2, Cistus, Copaiba, Cypress, Lavender, Palmarosa, Petitgrain

REPRODUCTIVE SYSTEM: PMS, menopause, pregnancy and labor, sexual frigidity, anxiety during labor and childbirth, low libido. APPLICATION: Personal inhaler, body oil, roll-on. PAIRS WITH: Lavender, Mandarin, Sweet Orange, Petitgrain, Ylang Ylang

PSYCHE/EMOTIONS: Depression, anxiety, heartache, agitation, tachycardia, insomnia, stress and stress-related conditions, panic attacks, hot, agitated conditions of the heart characterized by restlessness. APPLICATION: Personal inhaler, roll-on, body oil, cream, lotion, facial oil, aromatic bath. PAIRS WITH: Angelica Root, Bergamot Mint, Coriander Seed, Grapefruit, Mandarin, Sweet Orange, Petitgrain, Pinyon Pine, Valerian, Ylang Ylang

PALMAROSA

Palmarosa (*Cymbopogon martinii*, Poaceae) essential oil is steam distilled using the palmarosa grass. With its strong affinity to the skin, palmarosa supports the skin's health by promoting cellular rejuvenation and defends against bacterial or fungal infections.

SAFETY: No known contraindications

AROMA: Sweet, floral, rosy

SYSTEM AFFINITIES: Skin

BLENDS WELL WITH: Himalayan Cedarwood, Clove, Lavender, Laurel, Niaouli, Neroli, Rosemary ct. verbenone, Thyme ct. linalool

POTENTIAL SUBSTITUTIONS: Neroli

THERAPEUTIC APPLICATIONS

SKIN: Acne, dry skin, mature skin, fungal infections, dermatitis, eczema (dry and weeping), psoriasis, boils, wounds, cuts, wrinkles, itchy skin, broken capillaries. **APPLICATION:** Cleanser, cream or lotion, gel, body oil, salve, salt scrub Used in homemade underarm deodorant to prevent odor. **PAIRS WITH:** Himalayan Cedarwood, Lavender, Niaouli, Neroli, Rosemary ct. verbenone, Thyme ct. linalool

PSYCHE/EMOTIONS: Restlessness, anxiety, tension, nervous exhaustion, heartache, irritability, stress. **APPLICATION:** Personal inhaler, diffuser, roll-on. **PAIRS WITH:** Himalayan Cedarwood, Lavender, Neroli

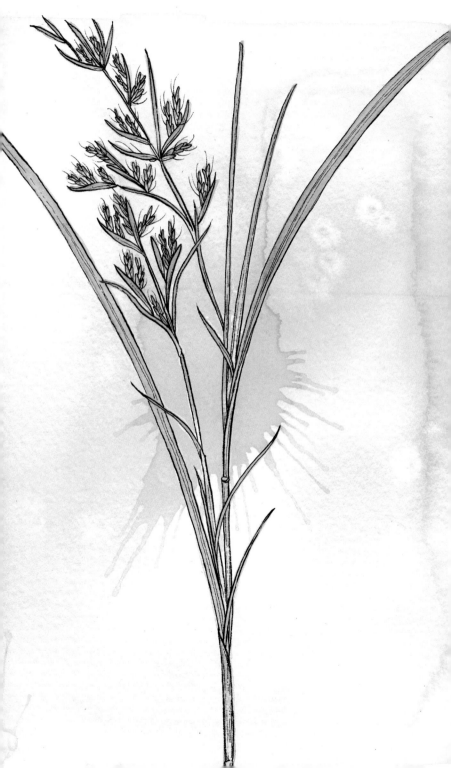

PATCHOULI

Patchouli (*Pogostemon cablin*, Lamiaceae) essential oil is steam distilled using dried patchouli leaves. People seem to either love or hate patchouli. It offers wonderful benefits for the skin due to its slightly astringent-like activity and skin soothing properties. Its aroma nourishes and calms the spirits (at least, it does if you love it!)

SAFETY: No known contraindications

AROMA: Strong, musty, earthy, dry

SYSTEM AFFINITIES: Skin

BLENDS WELL WITH: Angelica Root, Bergamot, Black Pepper, Cistus, Clary Sage, Cypress, Ginger, Grapefruit, Lavender, Lemongrass, Mandarin, Sweet Orange, Peppermint, Rose, Blue Tansy, Valerian

POTENTIAL SUBSTITUTIONS: Vetiver, Cypress

THERAPEUTIC APPLICATIONS

SKIN: Aging or sagging skin, itchy or inflamed skin conditions, acne, athlete's foot, cracked or chapped skin, eczema (weeping), wrinkles, irritated skin conditions, sores, allergic inflammation, cellulite. **APPLICATION:** Facial or body oil, body butter, aromatic gel, salves, salt scrubs. **PAIRS WITH:** Cistus, Cypress, Grapefruit, Lavender, Sweet Orange, Rose, Blue Tansy

REPRODUCTIVE SYSTEM: Frigidity, menstrual cramps, reduced or lack of sex drive, impotence. **APPLICATION:** Personal inhaler, body oil, diffuser, abdominal oil. **PAIRS WITH:** Bergamot, Black Pepper, Clary Sage, Grapefruit, Lavender, Mandarin, Sweet Orange, Rose

PSYCHE/EMOTIONS: Anxiety, depression, confusion, poor concentration, mood swings, hyperactivity, anxiety, feelings of being overwhelmed. **APPLICATION:** Body oil, body butter, salve (used like perfume), aromatic bath, unscented cream/lotion, personal inhaler, aromatic spritzer. **PAIRS WITH:** Angelica Root, Bergamot, Black Pepper, Clary Sage, Cypress, Grapefruit, Lavender, Mandarin, Sweet Orange, Rose, Valerian.

GENERAL: Useful in mosquito repellents, serves to hold other essential oils (as a base or fixative) so insect repellants and perfumes last longer and are more effective. **APPLICATION:** Aromatic spritzer. **PAIRS WITH:** Himalayan Cedarwood, Lemongrass, Peppermint

YARROW

Yarrow (*Achillea millefolium*, Asteraceae) essential oil is steam distilled using the flowering yarrow plant (feathery leaves and flowers). Yarrow is much loved for its wound healing and anti-inflammatory activity.

SAFETY: No known cautions

AROMA: Sweet, spicy, warm, fresh

SYSTEM AFFINITIES: Skin

BLENDS WELL WITH: Calendula CO_2, Cape Chamomile, German Chamomile, Roman Chamomile, Clary Sage, Cistus, Frankincense, Lavender, Neroli, Niaouli, Rosemary ct. verbenone

POTENTIAL SUBSTITUTIONS: Lavender, German Chamomile, Cape Chamomile

THERAPEUTIC APPLICATIONS

SKIN: Inflamed conditions, razor burn, dermatitis, acne, eczema, burns, cuts, rashes, scars, wounds, varicose veins, bruises. Tones the skin, slows bleeding from trauma, preventative to premature aging. **APPLICATION:** Cream, facial oil, cleanser, aromatic bath. **PAIRS WITH:** Cape Chamomile, Frankincense, Lavender, Calendula CO_2, Cistus, German Chamomile

MUSCULOSKELETAL SYSTEM: Arthritis, rheumatism, aches and pains, stiffness, cramps, tendinitis. **APPLICATION:** Body oil, gel, salve, lotion. **PAIRS WITH:** Clary Sage, Cape Chamomile, Lavender, Rosemary ct. cineole or Rosemary ct. camphor

PSYCHE/EMOTIONS: Nervous tension, irritability, neuralgia, insomnia, nervousness, anxiety, depression, restlessness. **APPLICATION:** Body butter, personal inhaler, aromatic bath, diffuser. **PAIRS WITH:** Cape Chamomile, Frankincense, Lavender, German Chamomile

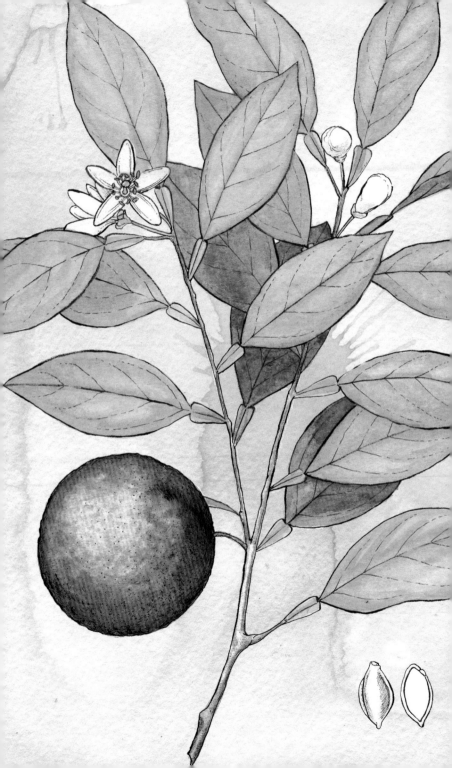

PETITGRAIN

Petitgrain (*Citrus aurantium* var. *amara*, Rutaceae) essential oil is steam distilled using the leaves of the bitter orange tree. Much loved for its stress-relieving aroma, petitgrain is used almost exclusively for emotional well-being and skin care.

DERMAL CAUTION: No known cautions or contraindications

AROMA: Woody, dry, floral, light

SYSTEM AFFINITIES: Nervous, psyche/emotions, skin

BLENDS WELL WITH: Cypress, Grapefruit, Lavender, Lemon, Mandarin, Sweet Marjoram, Neroli, Sweet Orange, Patchouli, Rose

POTENTIAL SUBSTITUTIONS: Lavender, Neroli, Bitter Orange

THERAPEUTIC APPLICATIONS

SKIN: Acne, inflamed skin (supports neroli and lavender), eczema, boils. A mild astringent, good for oily as well as dry skin, toning, wound healing. **APPLICATION:** Cleanser, gel, unscented cream. **PAIRS WITH:** Cypress, Grapefruit, Lavender, Lemon, Neroli, Patchouli, Rose

REPRODUCTIVE SYSTEM: Menstrual cramps, PMS, emotions associated with menopause. Could be used during childbirth as a pleasant, relaxing aroma. **APPLICATION:** Personal inhaler, abdominal oil, diffuser, nebulizing diffuser. **PAIRS WITH:** Cypress, Grapefruit, Lavender, Mandarin, Sweet Marjoram, Neroli, Sweet Orange, Patchouli, Rose

PSYCHE/EMOTIONS: Anxiety, tension, nervousness, irritation, insomnia, mental fatigue, mild depression, heart palpitations from anxiety or stress, agitation, psychological stress. **APPLICATION:** Personal inhaler, diffuser, roll-on, body oil, salt scrub, body butter. **PAIRS WITH:** Cypress, Grapefruit, Lavender, Lemon, Mandarin, Sweet Marjoram, Neroli, Sweet Orange, Patchouli, Rose

THYME

Thyme (*Thymus vulgaris*, Lamiaceae) essential oil has several chemotypes available. In this book we will focus on two of the main thyme chemotypes we find ourselves using on a regular basis.

THYME CT. LINALOOL

SAFETY: No known cautions or contraindications

AROMA: Sweet, slightly floral, soft herbaceous

SYSTEM AFFINITIES: Skin

BLENDS WELL WITH: Calendula CO_2, Roman Chamomile, Coriander

POTENTIAL SUBSTITUTIONS: Niaouli

THERAPEUTIC APPLICATIONS

SKIN: Skin infections, acne. **APPLICATION:** Gel, unscented cream or lotion, facial cleanser. **PAIRS WITH:** Roman Chamomile, Copaiba, Cypress

RESPIRATORY SYSTEM: Lowered immunity, respiratory infections. **APPLICATION:** Salve, steam inhalation. **PAIRS WITH:** Cypress, Blue Gum Eucalyptus, Inula, Laurel, Niaouli

MUSCULOSKELETAL SYSTEM: Muscular aches and pains, cramps, spasms, and rheumatic pain. **APPLICATION:** Salve, unscented cream or lotion, body oil. **PAIRS WITH:** Bergamot Mint, Black Pepper, Clary Sage, Lavender

THYME CT. THYMOL

DERMAL CAUTION: Potential mucus membrane irritant. Avoid use in baths or undiluted to avoid skin irritation.

AROMA: Sharp, herbaceous

SYSTEM AFFINITIES: Respiratory, digestive

BLENDS WELL WITH: Roman Chamomile, Cypress, Blue Gum Eucalyptus, Grapefruit, Inula, Laurel, Green Myrtle, Niaouli, Plai, Thyme ct. linalool

POTENTIAL SUBSTITUTIONS: Niaouli, Thyme ct. linalool

THERAPEUTIC APPLICATIONS

RESPIRATORY SYSTEM: Bronchitis, sinusitis, respiratory infections, coughs, colds, flu. Powerful anti-infectious essential oil. **APPLICATION:** Steam inhalation, personal inhaler, chest salve, chest oil. **PAIRS WITH:** Cypress, Blue Gum Eucalyptus, Inula, Laurel, Green Myrtle, Plai, Thyme ct. linalool

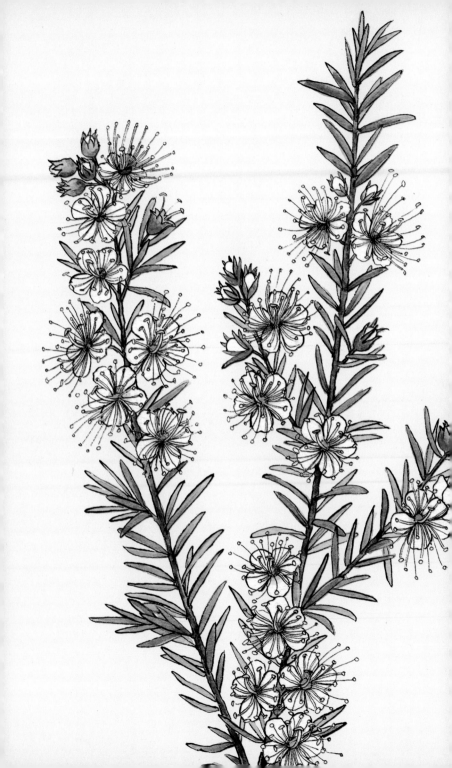

3

Expanding Your Apothecary

BEFORE WE DIVE into making body care products, we'll need to expand your apothecary with a few other botanical ingredients. Aromatherapy body care products are made up of essential oils and some type of base, such as a carrier oil and/or herbal oil, an unscented cream or lotion, or a gel or salve. The following chart outlines the ingredients that each body care product covered in this book may contain. The lowercase x stands for optional or dependent upon needs of product making.

	CO	HO	HY	WX	BT	AO
Body and Facial Oils	X	X				X
Roll-On (aka Roller Balls)	X	X				
Body Butters	X	X			X	X
Aromatic Gels	X	X	X			
Salves	X	X		X	X	X
Lip Balm	X	X		X	X	
Salt Scrubs	X	X				

Key to Codes

CO Carrier oil (includes vegetable oils and specialty seed oils, e.g., rosehip seed, borage)

HO Herbal oils (e.g., Calendula, St. John's Wort, Arnica)

HY Hydrosol(s)

WX Wax

BT Butter

AO Antioxidant

You can choose to make a body care product for its therapeutic benefits (e.g., a respiratory salve or salve to reduce inflamed skin conditions) or simply for the beauty and emotional support the aromatics provide (e.g., salve with rose, sweet orange, and patchouli used as a perfume).

Now let's add to your apothecary by understanding the ingredients needed to make various body care products.

Carrier Oils

Carrier oils, also commonly referred to as vegetable oils, are expeller pressed (using a type of pressing machine that extracts the oil) from seeds, nuts, and whole fruits. They are called "carrier" oils because they help dilute and carry the essential oils onto the skin.

On their own, carrier oils have incredible therapeutic benefits that support the skin's health and vitality. Carrier oils contain a rich array of fat-soluble vitamins, fatty acids, and essential fatty acids that not only help nourish the skin, but also protect the skin's barrier function, protect and repair the skin from damage (be it from the sun or free radicals), and prevent transepidermal water loss (TEWL). Carrier oils can also support the tone, elasticity, shape, and resiliency of the skin.

CARRIER OILS AND THEIR PROPERTIES

The following chart provides information on a variety of carrier oils. Our favorite carrier oils and the ones we tend to use the most are: jojoba oil, sesame seed oil, and sunflower seed oil. These three carriers are readily available, relatively inexpensive, and can be used at 100 percent.

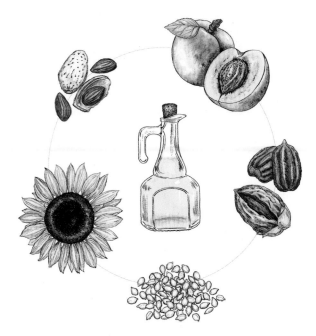

CARRIER OIL	PROPERTIES
AVOCADO OIL *Persea americana* **Shelf Life:** Up to 12 months. Can add mixed tocopherols or vitamin E to elongate shelf life: 0.04% to 1.0%.	Avocado oil offers powerful revitalizing and cell regenerative activity. Avocado is a wonderful emollient with great penetration. It's indicated specifically for maturing skin and dry skin. Postmenopausal skin, dry, dehydrated, fragile, or mature skin, and premature aging symptoms would all benefit from avocado oil. **Use:** 10 to 15% dilution of the total carrier oil amount
BAOBAB OIL *Adansonia digitata* **Shelf Life:** 2 to 4 years dependent upon the conditions of storage. Extremely stable oil.	Baobab oil is a heavier oil than most other carrier oils, with great emollient qualities for the skin supporting the skins' barrier function and lipid matrix while preventing water loss. **Use:** 25 to 100% dilution of the total carrier oil amount

CARRIER OIL	PROPERTIES
BORAGE SEED OIL *Borago officinalis* **Shelf Life:** Once opened, up to 6 to 9 months dependent upon the conditions of storage. **EVENING PRIMROSE OIL** *Oenothera biennis* **Shelf Life:** Once opened, up to 12 months dependent upon the conditions of storage.	Borage seed oil and Evening primrose oil are used for preventing premature aging of the skin as well as for regenerative skin care. Both oils also reduce inflammation and are used for psoriasis, eczema, and atopic dermatitis. **Use:** 10 to 25% dilution of the total carrier oil amount
JOJOBA OIL *Simmondsia chinensis* **Shelf Life:** Once opened, up to 12 to 24 months dependent upon the conditions of storage.	What's most fascinating about this oil is that its molecular structure resembles a liquid wax rather than a lipid-rich oil. Because of its chemical composition, our skin finds it familiar to our own sebum, and subsequently it is quite effective when applied to soothe inflammation, support resiliency, and bring the skin back into balance. Jojoba helps oily skin, particularly if pores are clogged and/or inflamed. It's fast absorbing and stable. Jojoba is highly versatile and can be a central ingredient in a wide array of skin and body care products. It is quite lovely when infused with vanilla beans. There are a lot of recipes on the internet.
NEEM OIL *Azadirachta indica* **Shelf Life:** Once opened, up to 6 to 9 months dependent upon the conditions of storage.	Native to India, Neem oil has a very potent pungent diffusive aroma. The oil shines in its ability to address dandruff, dry itchy scalps, and dry, damaged hair. Neem oil is also used in body care products for acne, eczema, foot fungus, and oily skin. Neem oil also has mosquito-repellent qualities. **Use:** 10 to 100% dilution of the total carrier oil amount

→

CARRIER OIL	PROPERTIES
POMEGRANATE OIL AND CO_2 TOTAL EXTRACT *Punica granatum* **Shelf Life:** Once opened, up to 6 to 9 months dependent upon the conditions of storage.	Pomegranate oil and CO_2 total extract soothes dermal inflammations such as acne, sunburn, psoriasis, and rosacea. It supports cellular regeneration, is a great antioxidant, improves skin elasticity, revitalizes prematurely aging or sun damaged skin, and is an incredibly beneficial emollient for dry skin conditions. **Carrier oil:** 10 to 15% dilution of the total carrier oil amount **CO_2 total extract:** 1 to 15%
ROSEHIP SEED OIL AND CO_2 TOTAL EXTRACT *Rosa canina* or *Rosa rubignosa* **Shelf Life:** Once opened, up to 6 to 9 months dependent upon the conditions of storage.	Rosehip seed oil and CO_2 total extract are most often used for supporting cellular rejuvenation and preventing premature aging of the skin. Either can be added to body care formulations for wound healing, to reduce age spots, and for regenerative skin care (tissue regeneration). Postmenopausal, dry, dehydrated, fragile, mature, and prematurely aging skin would all benefit from rosehip seed oil and total CO_2 extract. **Carrier oil:** 10 to 50% dilution of the total carrier oil amount **CO_2 total extract:** 1 to 15%
SEA BUCKTHORN OIL *Hippophae rhamnoides* **Shelf Life:** Once opened, up to 6 to 9 months dependent upon the conditions of storage.	Sea buckthorn's vibrant orange colored carrier oil and CO_2 total extract are used to support healing of the skin, reduce inflammation with conditions such as eczema or psoriasis. This oil supports wound healing, slow or poorly healing wounds, and healing the skin from sun damage. **Carrier oil:** 5 to 10% dilution of the total carrier oil amount **CO_2 total extract:** 1 to 15% **Note:** Due to sea buckthorn's rich orange color, it can stain clothing and other material it comes into contact with. Rinse material in cold soapy water immediately to remove oil.

CARRIER OIL	PROPERTIES
SESAME OIL *Sesamum indicum* **Shelf Life:** Up to 24 months. Sesame is one of the oils most resistant to oxidation because it contains the powerful natural antioxidants sesamolin and sesamin.	Sesame is also used to protect our skin from free-radical damage, and it strengthens the resiliency of our skin's barrier function with its trace vitamins and minerals. It has an oilier feel to the skin than jojoba and a very slight sesame-like aroma.
SUNFLOWER OIL *Helianthus annuus* **Shelf Life:** Once opened, up to 12 months dependent upon the conditions of storage.	Sunflower oil serves as a base oil that readily receives other more therapeutic carriers such as rosehip seed, calendula herbal oil, pomegranate seed oil. **Note:** Sunflower is available as both an oleic-rich and linoleic-rich oil. Here we are discussing the use of the oleic-rich sunflower oil, which is most commonly available due to its stability even when exposed to heat.
TAMANU OIL *Calophyllum inophyllum* **Shelf Life:** Once opened, up to 6 to 9 months dependent upon the conditions of storage.	Tamanu oil is a rich, aromatic carrier oil with a wide range of applications, many of which are based upon its traditional uses. Native to Southeast Asia, the tamanu tree is also found in Thailand, Vietnam, Myanmar, Malaysia, South India, and Sri Lanka. Tamanu is cell regenerative, wound healing, supportive to healthy scar tissue formation, and anti-inflammatory. It is also incredibly beneficial for dry/scaly skin conditions (e.g., psoriasis). **Use:** 10 to 100% dilution of the total carrier oil amount

Herbal Oils

An herbal oil is made by combining plant material (e.g., dried calendula flowers) with a vegetable oil, typically extra virgin olive oil or oleic-rich sunflower oil, and allowing the plant material to soak in the oil for up to 3 months. During that time, the vegetable oil absorbs fat-soluble components from the plant material, many of which have therapeutic activity beneficial to the skin, muscles, and joints.

One of the herbal oils most commonly used in aromatherapy products is **Calendula** (*Calendula officinalis*). Calendula herbal oil soothes dry or inflamed skin, and it supports healing of mild burns, insect bites, and wounds. Calendula herbal oil also simply supports the health of the skin and can be used in facial oils, creams, lotions, and even gels.

St. John's wort (*Hypericum perforatum*) herbal oil is used in body care products such as gels or salves for insect bites, bruises, muscle pain, and inflamed skin conditions. St. John's wort helps reduce inflammation and relieve pain.

Arnica (*Arnica montana*) herbal oil is used to relieve pain, support microcirculation, and reduce inflammation. Arnica herbal oil is used in body oils, salves, and homemade creams and lotions (designed for application to a localized area, e.g., the knees or wrists). Arnica oil is used for bruises, arthritis, bursitis, myalgia, sprains and strains, joint stiffness, and varicose veins. Safety note: Arnica herbal oil should not be applied to broken or damaged skin.

Plant-derived Butters

Butters provide a nutrient-dense component to essential oil-focused skin care recipes indicated for damaged, weakened, and stressed skin. Butters are used in lip balms and body butters in this book. However, you may also see them used in homemade cream and lotion recipes. Butters such as shea, mango, and illipe have a remarkable capacity to heal tissue, soften the skin, strengthen the skin's barrier function, and prevent transepidermal water loss, thus preventing or healing dry skin.

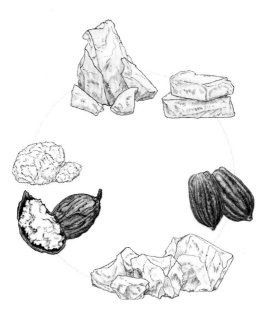

The two most commonly used plant-based butters for aromatherapy body care products are shea butter and cocoa butter. They're used for slightly different purposes. Let's explore.

Shea butter (*Vitellaria paradoxa* syn. *Butyrospermum parkii*), extracted from the African shea nut tree, is softer to the touch than cocoa butter, and shares many of its therapeutic benefits. Shea butter softens and soothes dry, damaged skin and can relieve skin irritation. It can support tissue regeneration and resiliency. However, shea butter is commonly used in and of itself for making whipped or regular body butters. Cocoa butter could not be used by itself to make a body butter, but it can be added in smaller amounts to support the therapeutic benefits of the butter. Unrefined shea butter is light to darker yellow in color and has a nutty, earthy aroma. Shea butter is used in body butters, lip balms, body balms, and at times, salves. It can be used up to 25 to 100% of a body butter or in a homemade cream or lotion. The shelf life of shea butter is 12 to 24 months when stored correctly.

Cocoa butter (*Theobroma cacao*) is the natural fatty byproduct of making chocolate from cocoa beans. Cocoa butter is used in lip balms, body butters, and homemade creams and lotions, and will harden in any product made with it. Due to its thickening/hardening nature, cocoa butter is used in low amounts. It can support the skin's health and prevent water loss—hence the reason why it is used in lip balms! It is recommended to use about 20 to 35 percent of the total recipe/formulation for body butters.

Unrefined cocoa butter smells strongly of chocolate, and it can often overpower the aromas of essential oils that are blended into it. We recommend choosing essential oils that smell good paired with the light scent of chocolate. Cocoa butter can last up to 2 to 5 years when stored properly. Keep away from heat, sunlight, and air. Note: Avoid over-heating cocoa butter. Overheating or heating for too long breaks chemical bonds within the cocoa butter, resulting in its inability to harden again.

Waxes

For aromatherapy body care products, there are two core waxes to choose from: beeswax and a vegan alternative, candelilla wax. Wax is used in lip balms, salves, and homemade creams and lotions. It is used to thicken the product and is typically used at between 10 percent and 25 percent of the total recipe, depending on the product being made.

Beeswax is typically a rich golden color, but it can vary depending on the propolis and colors within the pollen bees carry back to the hive. Beeswax has a beautiful sweet, honey-like aroma, which it imparts gently to the body care products that contain it. Please note: Bees and other pollinating insects face challenges in the ecosystems in which they play an essential role. If and when possible, purchase your beeswax from a local beekeeper, who uses healthy, sustainable practices.

Candelilla wax is derived from the leaves of the small candelilla shrub, *Euphorbia cerifera* and *Euphorbia antisyphilitica*, which is native to northern Mexico and the southwestern United States. It is a yellowish-brown color and, like beeswax, is lightly aromatic. Candelilla wax is typically used at 10 to 12 percent of the total recipe.

Hydrosols: Aromatic Waters

Hydrosols, also known as hydrolats, are one of the products of the distillation process. Hydrosols are quickly becoming much beloved for their gentle yet exceptional benefits for the skin and on emotional well-being. Artisan distillers all over the world are producing small batch hydrosols from ethically wild-crafted indigenous plants or lovingly cultivated plants grown for hydrosol distillation. There's never been a better time to explore these remarkable healing waters.

Hydrosols can soothe irritation, clean away bacteria and microbes from a cut or injury, reduce inflammation, support wound healing, soothe a sunburn, soothe irritated skin, and be used in gels for the skin, muscular aches and pains, or varicose veins.

Hydrosols can be used in baths, aromatic spritzers, homemade creams and lotions, and cleansers. They can also be used as toners for gentle skin care.

How much hydrosol to use?

- **Baths**
  - » Infants: 1 teaspoon (5 ml) of chosen hydrosol to an infant bathtub
  - » Children 2 to 6 years: 1 teaspoon (5 ml) of hydrosol per year of age, up to a maximum of 2 to 8 teaspoons (10 to 40 ml)
  - » 7 years and above and adults: 1 to 9 ounces (30 to 250 ml) per tub

- **Foot bath** (ages 7 years and above): 2 to 4 tablespoons (30 to 60 ml)

- **Aromatic Spritzers**: 10 to 100 percent of the total

- **Toners:** 50 to 100 percent of the total

- **Homemade creams and lotions:** Use for water portion of recipe

- **Cleansers:** approximately 1 teaspoon (5 ml) per ounce (28 ml) of liquid castile soap

To keep hydrosols fresh, it is important to keep them cool and away from direct light or heat. The average shelf life for most hydrosols is 12 to 24 months. Store hydrosols in a cool room or in the fridge to ensure freshness, stability, and liveliness of aroma. Stable, they can last up to 2 years.

OUR FAVORITE HYDROSOLS

Calendula (*Calendula officinalis*): Calendula hydrosol is the best when it comes to having a first aid kit hydrosol, although using it with lavender or helichrysum hydrosols would make it even better. Prized for its wound healing, skin soothing, and antiseptic properties, calendula hydrosol can be used in gels or by itself for first aid. Spray on insect bites, mild cuts and scrapes, sunburns, and other inflamed skin conditions.

Clary sage (*Salvia sclarea*): If ever there were a hydrosol for women of all ages, clary sage hydrosol would be it. Offering a powerful feminine energy, it can be spritzed into the air, used in a nourishing foot bath or full body bath, or sprayed on one's pillow after a long stressful day.

Rose geranium (*Pelargonium graveolens* var. *roseum*): Rose geranium hydrosol, like its essential oil, offers balance to the skin and the mind. Slightly astringent, rose geranium is indicated for oily skin conditions and can be beneficial as a toner for acne. The aroma calms and soothes the emotions.

German chamomile (*Matricaria chamomilla* syn. *Matricaria recutita*): German chamomile is an amazing hydrosol for cooling inflamed conditions, including emotional states such as irritability and anger. It's soothing for children and infants, whom it can help to fall asleep. Its ability to soothe inflamed skin conditions makes it a beneficial addition to a gel for applying to a sunburn.

Helichrysum (*Helichrysum italicum*): Helichrysum is a wonderful hydrosol for wound healing, both physical and emotional. Aromatic sprays using helichrysum can be applied directly to a cut or burn to help keep the wound clean and to support the wound healing process. Helichrysum reduces inflammation and supports cellular regeneration.

Lavender (*Lavandula angustifolia*): Lavender, along with German chamomile, are our go-to hydrosols for infants and young children as well as the skin. Sprayed into the air, lavender hydrosol can calm emotions and prepare young ones for bed. It could also be used in a water-based diffuser to lightly scent the air for a good night's sleep. Lavender hydrosol can also be used in infant baths or as a linen spray.

Neroli, also called orange flower (*Citrus aurantium* var. *amara*): beautiful and floral, slightly astringent, yet expansively compassionate and gentle, Neroli hydrosol is a great facial toner for oily skin types or for those who are being emotionally affected by the appearance, however transitional, of their skin. Neroli hydrosol's aroma is like a warm sunshine embrace.

Rose (*Rosa* × *damascena*): Rose hydrosol is much loved for its beautiful aroma and gentleness to the heart and skin. It is a wonderful hydrosol for oily skin as well as for bug or insect bites, mild cuts and scrapes, and heat rash from the sun. Aromatically, rose hydrosol sprayed into the air can calm and soothe the heart, relieve tension, and nourish the mind.

Witch hazel (*Hamamelis virginiana*): Witch hazel is often sold at pharmacy stores and is diluted down with rubbing alcohol. And although it is still used for cleaning wounds and supporting tissue healing, the hydrosol, in and of itself, is also used for bug or insect bites, mild cuts and scrapes, cleansing mild wounds, and reducing heat rash. Unlike other hydrosols, witch hazel hydrosol (without alcohol) has a shelf life of 8 to 12 months.

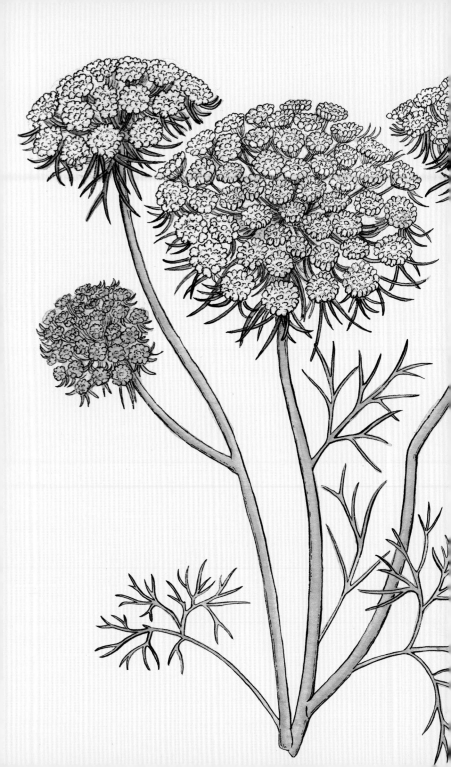

Body Care Applications

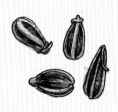

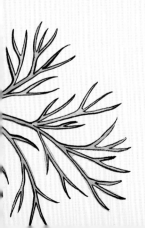

PERHAPS THE MOST amazing thing about essential oils is that there are so many ways in which to use them. In this chapter, we will explore the most popular ways to integrate them into your life, wellness apothecary, and home.

Body and Facial Oils

Making your own body or facial oil is a great way to enjoy the benefits of aroma while also supporting the health of your skin and body! Body oils not only nourish the skin, they are beneficial for relieving stress, providing pain relief, and relieving muscle spasms or cramps. You can also relieve tension in the neck and upper back from sitting at a computer all day by applying an aromatic body oil to that area. Body oils can also be used for massage. If you are planning a visit to a massage therapist, consider asking them to use a massage oil you made yourself.

Facial oils, on the other hand, are specifically designed to nourish the facial skin. Facial oils will often contain special carrier oils such as rosehip seed oil, sea buckthorn, and calendula herbal oil.

WHAT YOU NEED
- Essential oils
- Carrier oil(s)
- Herbal oil(s)
- Antioxidant, if using rosehip seed or other omega-3 rich vegetable oils
- Bottle; use either a glass bottle with phenolic cap or a PET bottle
  - » For facial oils, we recommend making up 1 fluid ounce (30 ml) at a time
  - » For body oils, we recommend 2 to 4 fluid ounces (60 to 120 ml) at a time

- Glass measuring cup
- Blank label

SHELF LIFE: 6 to 12 months from the time the product is made. However, we recommend using handmade products up within a three- to six-month period. We believe that once blended into a carrier oil, the aromatics begin to slowly age. As they age, they begin to lose their vitality.

PROCEDURE

1. Decide how much oil you will be making.

2. Select one to three essential oils to be used for a blend.

3. Select carrier oil(s).

4. Measure your ingredients depending on the dilution:
   - » For body oils, you will need a total of 15 to 20 drops of essential oil per fluid ounce (30 ml).
   - » For facial oils, you will need a total of 7 to 14 drops per fluid ounce (30 ml).

5. Place all essential oil drops in the bottle. Swivel or shake the bottle.

6. Pour in carrier oil(s). Cap tightly and shake until well combined.

7. Name your oil blend and label the bottle with its name and ingredients. Be sure to put the date when the product was made!

Roll-On (aka Roller Balls)

We love these roll-on bottles! The roller ball is basically a 0.35-ounce (10 ml) bottle with a cap or lid that contains a ball. They're not only useful for application, they make great holiday gifts for your friends.

Each roller bottle holds 0.3 ounce (9 ml) of base oil. Choose what you have in stock: jojoba, sesame, rosehip seed, calendula herbal oil, or the like. Base oils add nourishment and may add color and/or an aroma. The possibilities are endless.

The average number of drops of essential oils to use is between 5 and 12, depending on which are being used and the goal of your roller ball formulation. For example, you could use less of essential oils such as rose or more of monoterpene-rich essential oils, such as the conifers or citrus essential oils.

PROCEDURE

It helps to have small beakers, such as in 1.75 ounces (50 ml) or 3.5 ounces (100 ml) sizes, on hand, but a small measuring cup works too.

1. Fill beaker with the carrier oil of your choice.

2. Pour oil into the bottle, just to the lip (where the side begins to turn in and go up). You don't want to fill it up to the very top!

3. Add in your drops of essential oil(s).

4. Holding a clean fingertip over the top, shake the bottle vigorously.

5. Smell the final blend to make sure it smells the way you would like it to. Adjust as necessary.

6. Place the ball and cap onto the inside lid.

7. Place the cap on the bottle.

8. Label the bottle. It's ready to be used.

TO MAKE A BATCH OF 10 AROMATHERAPY ROLLER BALLS

1. Measure 3 fluid ounces (90 ml) of base oil(s).

2. Measure 70 drops of essential oil synergy (see page 142) or a single essential oil.

3. Combine essential oil synergy with carrier oil.

4. Stir with a metal or glass stir rod until well combined.

5. Pour blend into each bottle, filling just to where the lip begins to turn up.

6. Pop ball/lids into bottles. Cap.

7. Place a label on each bottle.

8. Give to friends and family!

Body Butters

Body butters provide a nutrient-dense product to help heal and soothe damaged, weakened, or stressed skin. They have the remarkable capacity to heal tissue, soften dry areas of skin such as the elbows, knees, or feet, and perhaps most importantly, protect the skin's barrier function by preventing water loss. Body butters are most commonly used for dry, itchy skin conditions (where itchiness is caused by dryness) and to protect the skin from moisture loss, such as during the winter months when our skin is dealing with the cold and windy weather along with heat inside our living and working areas.

Body butters are made utilizing natural butters along with at least one carrier and/or herbal oil. Body butters do not contain water, so they do not need a preservative. However, depending on which vegetable oils you use in your formulation, you may want to consider adding in 1 percent antioxidant such as rosemary CO_2 extract, vitamin E, or mixed tocopherols.

WHAT YOU NEED
- A butter (e.g., shea butter) that is not cocoa; cocoa butter is not used to make body butters except when added in a low percentage to avoid making the butter too hard.
- Essential oils
- Carrier oil(s)
- Herbal oil(s)

SHELF LIFE:
- Most butters are good for up to 6 to 12 months.
- Depending on which base oils you choose, you may consider adding in 1 percent vitamin E or 0.5 to 1 percent rosemary CO_2 extract. We recommend adding one of these antioxidants to a body butter when using vegetable oils such as flax, rosehip seed, evening primrose, or borage.

Aromatic Gels

Aromatic gels are used for insect bites, bruises, sunburns, small burns, and muscular aches and pains (e.g., shoulders and neck area), on the temples to soothe headaches, and to soothe inflamed or irritated skin. Gels are cooling by nature. The most commonly used gel for making aromatherapy products is aloe vera gel. Aloe vera gel has a long history of use in treating simple burns, including sunburn. Aloe vera gel may also be used to make homemade hand sanitizers.

PREP TIME: 30 minutes

YIELD: varies

SHELF LIFE: Store gels in a cool room or fridge. Unpreserved gels or gels made with commercial aloe vera gel or gelly (which do have a basic preservative system) can last up to 1 to 3 months. With gels, it is a good idea to make up only a small amount, approximately 2 to 4 ounces (60 to 120 ml) at a time.

WHAT YOU NEED
- Essential oils
- Aloe vera gel or gelly
- Hydrosols

PROCEDURE
1. Select one to three essential oils.

2. Measure out a total of 10 to 15 drops of essential oil per ounce (30 ml) of aloe vera gel into a small bowl.

3. Measure aloe vera gel into the bowl.

4. Stir with a stainless steel spoon or fork until well combined.

5. Scoop gel out of the bowl into a clean jar.

6. Label, being sure to list the ingredients.

7. Use as needed. Store in a cool area.

Salves

If you have ever used Vicks VapoRub, then you have used a type of salve. Aromatic salves are made up of beeswax, vegetable and/or herbal oils (e.g., Calendula), and essential oils. You can make salves thicker by simply adding more beeswax or semisolid by adding less beeswax. It's up to you!

Why use a salve? Salves are amazing for congestion and for small localized applications for such things as insect bites and dry patches of skin.

PREP TIME: 60 minutes
YIELD: Two 1 oz (30 ml) jars and one 0.5 ounce (15 ml) jar
Safety: Salves should not be applied to poison ivy rashes, weepy eczema, pimples, boils, fresh sunburn, or fungal or bacterial skin infections.

WHAT YOU NEED
- Double boiler (stainless steel)
- Glass measuring cup
- Small scale to weigh beeswax
- Tins or glass jars
- Stainless steel fork or stirring rod
- Paper towels

INGREDIENTS
- ¼ cup (60 ml) vegetable and/or herbal oil(s)
- ¼ oz (7 g) beeswax or candelilla wax
- 30 to 50 drops essential oils

PROCEDURE
1. Clean the space where you will be making salve.

2. Clean all utensils, the double boiler, and the bowls or measuring cups.

3. Fill the bottom pot of the double boiler with 2 to 3 cups (500 to 700 ml) of water. Place the top pan on the bottom pot. Place the double boiler onto medium heat and heat water to just below boiling.

4. Add in wax. Allow it to begin melting. Then add the carrier oils.

5. Stir ingredients together until well combined.

6. Once all the beeswax is melted, remove from heat and add in the essential oils.

7. Stir the essential oils quickly into the salve mixture.

8. Pour salve into jars or tins. If the salve begins to harden, place the pot back onto the double boiler (turn heat back on if necessary).

9. Place a cap on the jars or tins and allow the salve to harden.

10. Check salves to make sure you like the texture and that the aroma is of a desired strength based upon the purposes of the salve.

11. Create labels for your salve jars and include all the ingredients.

12. Once salves are labeled, they are ready to use!

NOTE: Test the consistency of a salve before blending it with other essential oils by placing a spoonful of the salve in the refrigerator. Allow it to harden. If the salve comes out too hard or thick, you can melt the mixture down again and add more oil. If the salve is too fluid or thin, you can melt it down and mix in some more beeswax.

DILUTION/DOSAGE RECOMMENDATION:
The salve-making dosage may seem a bit high, but this is because a salve holds essential oils differently than other delivery systems do. Our recommended dosage is 30 to 40 drops per ounce (30 g) of salve.

Salt Scrubs

We love salt scrubs. They stimulate circulation and remove dead skin cells while leaving the skin radiant. In creating a salt scrub, it is best to use a fine- to medium-sized sea salt. Epsom salt does not seem to work as well. Stay away from anything too coarse, as you don't want to scratch or damage the skin.

PREP TIME: 15 to 30 minutes

YIELD: This recipe will fill an 8-ounce (250 ml) jar.

Safety: Never apply salt scrub to broken skin. Salt can irritate the skin if used right after shaving or waxing. It's best to avoid salt scrubs for 24 to 48 hours after you do either.

WHAT YOU NEED

- 2 cups (540 g) sea salt
- ½ cup (120 ml) natural vegetable oil such as almond, apricot, or sunflower
- 7 to 25 drops essential oil(s), depending on the usage and strength desired

PROCEDURE

1. In a small bowl, mix sea salt and vegetable oil.

2. Add essential oils.

3. Stir until well combined.

TO USE

1. Wet the skin, either in the shower (then turn off the water) or by using a hydrosol or aromatic spritzer.

2. Apply the salt glow treatment to the desired area. Use quick, vigorous strokes or make it more relaxing with longer, slower strokes. The important thing is to keep the mixture and circulation moving.

3. Remove or rinse the mixture from the body by taking a warm shower.

4. Avoid using salt scrubs on the face, as this skin is too delicate and prone to scratching.

5. Be sure to conclude your salt glow with a natural moisturizing oil or lotion to feed and replenish the newly exfoliated skin.

Variations on the traditional salt glow can be achieved by incorporating dried herbs, ground nuts, seaweeds, and other natural ingredients.

Aromatic Baths

Bathing is a wonderful way to enjoy the beautiful aromas of essential oils while relaxing in warm water. Bathing with essential oils can reduce stress, emotional tension, and anxiety, and it can relieve muscular tension. Have trouble sleeping? Consider taking an evening aromatic bath with essential oils by candlelight.

PREP TIME: 5 to 15 minutes
YIELD: 1 bath
Safety: Avoid placing essential oils into the bath prior to getting into the bath. Do not use skin-irritating essential oils such as thyme, oregano, lemongrass, cinnamon bark or leaf or other phenol- or aldehyde-rich essential oils in the bath. Avoid using extra drops of essential oil. A few drops go a long way. Be cautious when using citrus or conifer essential oils. We recommend 2 to 3 drops for these essential oils.

WHAT YOU NEED
- Essential oil(s)
- Honey, liquid castile soap, solubol, glycerin, full-fat milk, vegetable oil, herbal oil, or another "dispersing" agent
- Small glass bowl (to blend in)

PROCEDURE
1. Add 3 to 7 drops of essential oil(s) into 1 tablespoon (30 ml) honey.

2. Once in the bath, gently pour the mixture into the bathwater. Use your fingers to remove any remaining product from the bowl.

Body and Facial Cleansers

Cleaning the skin is one of the most common rituals we have as humans. Who doesn't love to take a nice warm shower at the beginning or end of the day? The ritual of cleansing seems to provide one with a sense of rejuvenation. Body and facial cleansers are designed to remove dead skin cells, grime, excess sebum, stale makeup, sweat, and bacteria from the skin.

The most common cleanser used to make aromatherapy cleansers is liquid castile soap, an all-natural, vegetable-based cleansing product.

PREP TIME: 15 to 30 minutes

YIELD: Varies

SHELF LIFE: 6 to 12 months. However, we recommend using handmade products up within a 3- to 6-month period. We believe that once blended into a base, the aromatics will slowly begin to age and lose their vitality.

WHAT YOU NEED
- Essential oil(s)
- Unscented liquid castile soap (often available at a local natural health or grocery store). We recommend Dr. Bronner's Baby Unscented Pure-Castile Liquid Soap

PROCEDURE
1. Select one to three essential oils.

2. Add a total of 10 to 15 drops of essential oil per ounce (28 ml) of liquid castile soap.

3. Combine ingredients in a PET or glass bottle.

Creams and Lotions

Ever have dry skin? It's quite common, and it becomes even more common as we age due to changes in the skin. Other contributing factors to dry skin include lack of water and healthy fats in the diet. Make sure to cultivate a healthy diet that includes healthy fats and ensure you have good water intake throughout the day.

When it comes to aromatherapy and dry skin, creams and lotions are your best tools. They offer both oil and water to soften and soothe skin while supporting its ability to retain moisture. What's the difference between a cream and a lotion? Creams tend to be thicker than lotions and are commonly used on the face or on localized dry spots on the body. Lotions, on the other hand, tend to be thinner in texture and can be applied to the whole body.

The easiest way to incorporate essential oils into creams and lotions is to start with a cream or lotion on the market that you like and that works for your skin.

PREP TIME: 15 to 30 minutes

YIELD: Varies

SHELF LIFE: Most unscented creams and lotions commonly available in health food stores will have some type of preservative system. We recommend using cream or lotion up within 6 to 12 months. If using an unpreserved cream or lotion, the shelf life tends to be 1 to 6 months depending on how it is stored and used.

WHAT YOU NEED
- Unscented cream or lotion
- Essential oil(s)
- Bowl
- Spoon
- Silicone spatula

PROCEDURE

1. Select 3 to 5 essential oils (use an equal number of drops of each for the total number of recommended drops).

2. Measure and place the cream or lotion in a clean bowl.

3. Add in appropriate drops of each essential oil:
   - » Cream for face: 4 to 6 drops per ounce (30 ml); or
   - » Lotion: 7 to 14 drops per ounce (30 ml).

4. Stir the essential oil(s) into the cream or lotion using a stainless steel spoon. Stir until well combined.

5. Scoop the cream or lotion into a clean container.

6. Name the product, create a label, and place a label on jar. Be sure to list all the ingredients so you know what's in it.

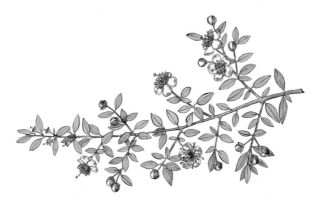

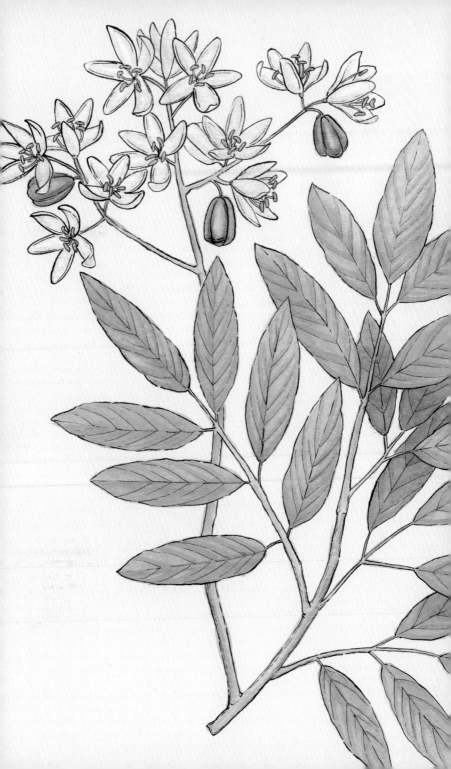

5

Diffusion and Inhalation

DIFFUSING ESSENTIAL OILS into the air or inhaling them is a great way to relieve stress and anxiety, support a good night's rest, increase alertness, improve air quality, and reduce airborne germs. While diffusion of essential oils tends to affect everyone within the environment being diffused, inhalation tends to be a personal interaction with the essential oils. With both diffusion and inhalation, you will be making a synergy of essential oils. A **synergy** is a combination of essential oils without a carrier/herbal oil or other base (e.g., cream, lotion, or gel). Synergies are designed to be used in diffusers (all types), in personal inhalers, or for steam inhalations.

You can also use hydrosols in some of the methods of application for diffusion and inhalation. See the chart below.

INHALATION/DIFFUSION		
	SY	HY
DIFFUSION		
Ultrasonic (water) diffuser	X	X
Candle diffuser	X	X
Nebulizing diffuser	X	
Aromatic spritzer	X	X
Personal inhaler	X	
Steam inhalation	X	X

Key to codes:

SY   Synergy: a combination of 3–5 essential oils without a base/carrier oil

HY   Hydrosol(s): also known as hydrolats, are one of the products of the distillation process

Diffusion

The most common tools used to diffuse essential oils into the environment are:

1. **Water diffuser, also known as an ultrasonic diffuser.** This type of diffuser uses an internal diaphragm that vibrates at ultrasonic frequency, which involves sound waves with a frequency above the upper limit of human hearing. This ultrasonic vibration turns the water into vapor, which carries essential oil molecules (aroma) into the atmosphere. These are great diffusers for smaller spaces in the home, such as a bedroom, home office, or living room. They are simple to use. Typically, add water to the bowl and add 5 to 10 drops of essential oil or synergy. Allow the diffuser to run for 15 to 30 minutes every hour.

2. **Candle diffuser.** Candle diffusers are a great way to benefit mood, energy, and other emotional states. Typically, candle diffusers are a piece of pottery designed with a small bowl on top and a place for a tealight candle underneath the bowl. The tealight gently warms the water in the bowl, which contains drops of an essential oil or a synergy of essential oils. The heating of the water slowly diffuses the aroma of the essential oil(s) used into the environment.

This is a beautiful way to enjoy the aroma of the essential oil(s) along with the ambience of a tealight, and it is simple to use. Fill the bowl with water and add 5 to 10 drops of an essential oil or synergy. Light the candle and place it underneath the bowl. Add more essential oil if needed. Allow the diffuser to go until the water is almost gone.

SAFETY:
- Do not leave a candle diffuser unattended.
- Keep a lit candle out of the reach of children.
- **Clean regularly with hot soapy water. Dry the unit, and then wipe with a paper towel and a bit of rubbing alcohol. You don't want mold growing in there!**

3. **Nebulizing diffuser.** This is an electric diffuser typically made out of three pieces: the base (a kind of pump that will blow air into the glass "nebulizer"), the glass nebulizer, and a small piece of glass that is placed onto the nebulizer to direct microdroplets of essential oil into the atmosphere. These microdroplets are suspended in the air for a short while.

This type of diffuser tends to be used in more clinical settings or by aromatherapy practitioners, although it can certainly be used in the home as well. The nebulizing diffuser is often the most expensive option for diffusing essential oils into the environment.

To clean the diffuser, soak the glass part in a solution of 70 percent alcohol or 100 percent rubbing alcohol or even vodka, for a few hours. Rinse with hot water and allow to dry completely before the next use.

USAGE AND SAFETY:
- Nebulizing diffusers are designed to be used 10 to 15 minutes every hour or 30 minutes every two hours. Do not run them continuously!
- Avoid the use of viscous essential oils such as vetiver, as these oils may clog the unit and can get a bit gummy, making them difficult (though not impossible) to remove. Use the cleaning method described above and soak it for a longer time. We have also found that using lemongrass essential oil can be beneficial in removing gummy stuff from glassware.
- Avoid using expensive essential oils such as melissa or rose. There are other less expensive essential oils with similar properties to diffuse.
- Do not use vegetable or other carrier oils in a nebulizing diffuser.

Aromatic Spritzers

Aromatic spritzers, also known as room sprays or linen sprays, have become popular for their ability not only to freshen and cleanse the air but also to uplift, relax, or energize those who are exposed to their aromas. Aromatic spritzers can also be used to reduce yucky odors in the air or to "scent" clothing, bed linens, and fabric on furniture.

The basic ingredients of aromatic spritzers are water (can use hydrosols 100 percent) and essential oils. We recommend using distilled water when possible and affordable. It not, tap water is fine too. For home use, water is fine, but you could also use vodka as the base for the spritzer. Or if you happen to have 190 proof grain alcohol hanging around, you could dilute it with water to 70 percent and use this as your base. The benefit of using 70 percent alcohol is that essential oils are soluble into the alcohol and no emulsifier would be needed. What is an emulsifier? An emulsifier is something that helps disperse essential oils into the water and reduces the need to shake the product with each use. Although beneficial if you're making a product line for retail sale, this is really unnecessary for home use and only adds to the cost of the spritzer.

YIELD: Depends on the size of the bottle (2 to 8 ounces [60 to 240 ml] is what we recommend)

PREP TIME: 30 minutes

SHELF LIFE: If made with distilled water only, 1 to 3 months when stored in a cool place. If made with 70 percent alcohol (and 30 percent water), store 6 to 12 months. We recommend using aromatic spritzers within 6 months if possible. This ensures the vitality of the aroma.

WHAT YOU NEED
- Spritzer bottle: We recommend a 2 to 8 ounce (60 to 240 ml) round glass or PET bottle with a spritzer top
- Distilled water (available at grocery stores) or hydrosols
- Optional: vodka or 190 proof alcohol diluted down to 70 percent alcohol/30 percent water
- Optional: emulsifier such as Solubol

1. Select one to three different, complementary essential oils, or a premade synergy.

2. Add a total of 10 to 15 drops of essential oil per ounce (30 ml) of water in a spritzer bottle. If using more than one essential oil, use equal drops of each to add up to 10 to 15 total drops.

3. Swivel the bottle to combine the oils.

4. Add distilled water or other chosen liquid.

5. Shake well prior to each use.

Personal Inhaler Tubes

Personal inhaler tubes can be used to relieve stress, uplift mood, reduce or relieve nausea (e.g., travel nausea), support emotional well-being, reduce sinus congestion, and provide support during challenging times.

Inhaler tubes are designed using 100 percent essential oil(s) saturated on a cotton pad. A personal inhaler is a fun and easy product to make and a safe method of application, so you can enjoy your inhaler throughout the day.

PREP TIME: 15 to 30 minutes
YIELD: 1 inhaler tube
SHELF LIFE: 6 to 12 months

WHAT YOU NEED
- Essential oils
- Small glass bowl
- Spoon
- Empty inhaler tube, including tube, cap, and cotton pad

PROCEDURE
1. Select two or three essential oils.

2. Decide how many drops of essential oil to use. We recommend a total of 20 to 25 drops to saturate the cotton pad. Equally divide drops among your chosen essential oils.

3. Add drops to a bowl.

4. Drop the cotton pad into the bowl and, using the tip of the spoon, gently move the pad around to soak up the oil.

5. Pick up the pad with tweezers or your fingers and insert it into the inhaler tube.

6. Place the bottom onto the inhaler tube and lid onto the top of the tube.

7. Be sure to create a label for the inhaler with ingredients listed.

8. Create a name for the inhaler based upon its purpose or therapeutic goal (e.g., Relax Inhaler).

Smelling Salts

Making your own smelling salts is a great alternative to using the plastic personal inhalers. With growing concerns about the widespread use of plastic along with the challenges of disposing of it, we recommend you consider this as a wonderful way to enjoy the aromatic benefits of essential oils.

PREP TIME: 10 to 20 minutes
YIELD: 1 container of smelling salts
SHELF LIFE: 6 to 12 months

WHAT YOU NEED
- Essential oils
- Fine- or medium-grind sea salt or Epsom salt
- ⅓ ounce (10 ml) European dropper bottle or other suitable small lidded glass container

PROCEDURE

1. Create a synergy with a total of 20 to 30 drops utilizing three to five essential oils. Place it in the glass container.

2. Gently shake the bottle to combine the oils.

3. Pour salt into the bottle.

4. Place the lid on the bottle and shake vigorously to coat all the salt with the synergy of essential oils.

5. Create a label for the bottle with its ingredients.

6. Name the salts based on their purpose or therapeutic goal.

Steam Inhalation

When Amandine Peter, one of the senior instructors at our school, was a child, her mother would boil some water and then pour it into a bowl on the kitchen table for Amy and her sisters to do steam inhalations when they were congested or had a cold. Amy loved putting the towel over her head and breathing in the warm vapors of steam and a bit of Vicks VapoRub.

Steam inhalations are incredibly beneficial for loosening congestion in the nasal cavity, allowing mucus to be thinned and expelled by blowing the nose. Steam inhalations with essential oils may also be used for things such as sinusitis, to help relieve inflammation and open up the nasal passages.

Steam inhalation is one of the most effective methods of application when it comes to afflictions of the respiratory system. The steam carries active compounds from the essential oils directly into the nose and down to the lungs. It is also easy to prepare. The following recipe just requires water and essential oils.

PREP TIME: 15 minutes
YIELD: 1 steam inhalation treatment
SAFETY: Avoid irritating essential oils such as oregano, thyme ct. thymol, cinnamon bark or cinnamon leaf. Be cautious using

peppermint essential oil; use only 1 drop. Do not open your eyes while doing steam inhalation. Avoid steam inhalations for children under the age of 5 years.

WHAT YOU NEED
- 1 to 3 essential oils
- 4 cups (950 ml) water
- Cooking pot or kettle
- Bowl for hot water
- Towel

Some essential oils to consider include: Eucalyptus (either *Eucalyptus globulus* or *Eucalyptus radiata*), Thyme ct. linalool (*Thymus vulgaris*), Lemon (*Citrus limon*), Green Myrtle (*Myrtus communis*)

PROCEDURE
1. Select one to three essential oil(s).

2. Place water in a pot or kettle and bring it to a boil.

3. Pour boiling water into the bowl.

4. Prepare for inhalations by placing the towel around your shoulders.

5. Place 1 to 2 drops of each essential oil into the bowl. The total should equal between 3 and 5 drops.

6. Place the towel over your head, shut your eyes, and bend over the steam. Take 5 to 10 deep slow breaths in through the nose.

7. Once complete, if water is still hot, you can repeat steps 5 and 6.

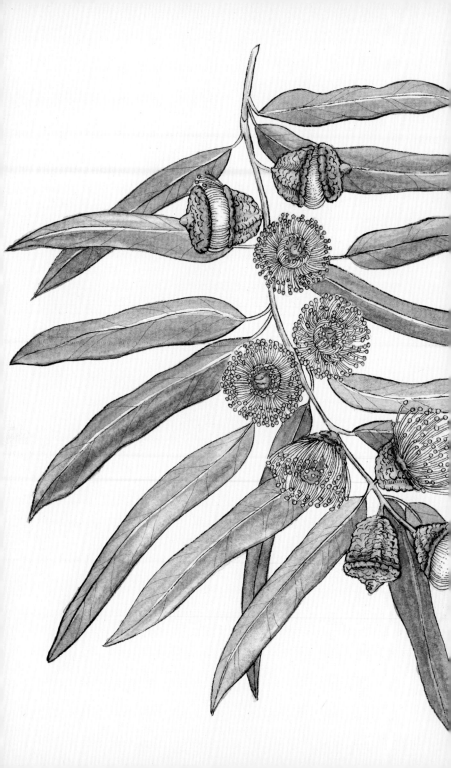

6

Blending Beyond Recipes

With so many recipes swirling around the internet and social media, it can be a bit overwhelming to try to tell which ones will really work for you—and expensive to experiment to find out! The answer to this conundrum: Learn how to create and make your own aromatherapy products, be they for your body or your health and wellness.

How to Formulate a Body Care Product

To begin formulating a body care product, answer the following questions.

1. **What product are you making?**

2. **What is the goal of the product?** To make a beautiful aromatic product? To make a therapeutic product for the skin? To create a synergy for supporting the respiratory system? Something else?

3. **Next, what ingredients make up the product?** Body care products contain a few other ingredients you will need to select when making your product. Here is the table of possible ingredients.

BODY CARE PRODUCTS	CO	HO	HY	WX
Body and Facial Oils	X	X		
Roll-On (aka Roller Balls)	X	X		
Body Butters	X	X		
Aromatic Gels	X	X	X	
Salves	X	X		X
Lip Balm	X	X		X
Salt Scrubs	X	X		
Unscented Cleansers			X	
Unscented Creams and Lotions	X	X	X	

Key to codes:

CO Carrier oils (includes vegetable oils and specialty seed oils; e.g., rosehip seed, borage)

HO Herbal oils (e.g., Calendula, St. John's wort, Arnica)

HY Hydrosol(s)

WX Wax

4. **How much are you making?**

5. **What is the best dilution rate for your product?** Refer to chart below. Typically, when making a body care product, your dilution will be between 1 and 2.5 percent.

DILUTION IN %	PURPOSE AND INDICATIONS
0	Essential oils should not be used for infants under 6 months of age unless absolutely necessary and only if one is trained to do so. Use hydrosols instead.
0.25% to 0.5%	Infants 6 months or older, frail or elderly individuals, immune compromised individuals.
1%	Children 2 to 5 years old.
1.5%	Subtle aromatherapy, emotional and energetic work, facial creams and lotions, exfoliants. Pregnant, frail, or elderly individuals.
2% to 5%	Action on the nervous system, emotional well-being, and response to daily stress. Holistic aromatherapy, general massage work, general skin care, massage oils, lotions, facial oils, body oils, and body butters.
7%	Treatment massage and localized treatment work, wound healing, body oils, butters, and salves.
10%	Muscular aches and pains, trauma injury, treatment massage, acute physical pain, localized treatment work, and salves.
Undiluted	Acute trauma. Use nonaggressive essential oils only.

And once you have your dilution rate chosen, you can figure out your drops using this chart.

	ESSENTIAL OIL DILUTION					
Carrier oil	0.5%	1%	2.5%	3%	5%	10%
½ ounce (15 ml)	1–3 drops	3–5 drops	8–11 drops	9–13 drops	15–23 drops	30–46 drops
1 ounce (30 ml)	3–5 drops	6–9 drops	15–23 drops	18–27 drops	30–45 drops	60–90 drops
2 ounces (60 ml)	6–10 drops	12–18 drops	30–46 drops	36–54 drops	60–90 drops	120–180 drops
4 ounces (118 ml)	12–20 drops	24–36 drops	60–92 drops	72–108 drops	120–180 drops	240–360 drops

How to Formulate a Synergy for a Diffuser or Inhalation

To begin formulating a synergy for a diffuser or inhalation, answer the following questions.

- **What is the goal for the synergy?** For example, "uplifting yet calming to stress synergy," or "citrusy."

- **Synergy ingredients:** Essential oils only.

- **Decide on the amount you will be making:** For example, 5- and 10-ml size bottles are two standard sizes for making a small batch of synergy.

1 ml = approx. 25 to 35 drops total of essential oil.

How to Select Essential Oils for a Synergy

Choosing three to five essential oils to work with requires a bit of practice. Once you have chosen how you are going to approach selecting them, you can then refer to the appropriate charts provided in this chapter to begin narrowing down your selection.

In our blending method, each essential oil we select serves a purpose toward the whole. We select our essential oils with the following approach:

- **The core essential oil.** The core essential oil is chosen based upon your primary purpose or goal and is considered the heart of the synergy.

- **The enhancer essential oil**. The enhancer essential oil strengthens the core essential oil in its purpose and therapeutic action.

- **The harmonizer essential oil.** The harmonizing essential oil supports and enhances the vitality and purpose of the overall synergy. The harmonizing essential oil often has a decisive impact on the overall aroma and is chosen for both its aroma and its ability to enhance the goals of the synergy.

- **Additional essential oils.** Optionally, you can decide to add one or two additional essential oils. This addition could be a core, enhancer, and/or harmonizer essential oil or essential oils. You decide!

There are a few ways to begin the selection process. On the next few pages are reference charts that have been designed to assist you in your selection.

These charts include:

1. **Aromatic Palette:** The tables provided in this palette are based upon different aromatic qualities, such as citrusy or forest. The aromatic palette provides a path of selecting essential oils based upon the aromatics desired. Let's say you would like to make an inhaler that is reminiscent of the forest; you could select fir, pine, and cypress from the forest palette. Or you could change the forest-only aroma to one that has a bit of citrus in in. Choose two essential oils from the forest palette and one from the citrus palette.

2. **Therapeutic:** The therapeutics chart categorizes essential oils based upon their affinities to different systems of the body. If you are seeking to make a respiratory remedy or a remedy that reduces menstrual cramps, this is the chart you will want to use.

3. **Morphology (Plant Part):** The morphology chart is based upon the energetic messages of the essential oil based upon the part of the plant it is derived from.

If approaching your product with emotions in mind, you may begin your search by using the aromatic palette or the morphology approach. If you are formulating a product or synergy for a health imbalance (e.g., respiratory congestion or sluggish digestion) then you can utilize the therapeutics chart.

Once you have selected the essential oils you would like to use in your product formulation, the next question before blending them together is:

DO THEY SMELL GOOD TOGETHER?

This is always done *before* blending them together. Remove the caps from all three to five bottles, place them together in your hands to ensure that all the bottle neck openings are the same height, and then waft the bottles under your nose.

What you want to notice is if the essential oils smell good together and if they appear to merge into one aroma as a group. If one essential oil seems to not merge very well with the others, you may decide to replace that one with another of similar aroma or therapeutic action. Whether blending for emotional/mental/spiritual or physical benefits, the essential oils should be complementary and supportive to one another in action and aroma.

AROMATIC PALETTES

FOREST AROMAS

Essential Oil	Latin name
Cedarwood	*Cedrus deodara*
Cedarwood, Virginia	*Juniperus virginiana*
Cypress	*Cupressus sempervirens*
Fir, Balsam	*Abies balsamea*
Juniper Berry	*Juniperus communis*
Pine, Scots	*Pinus sylvestris*
Pinyon Pine	*Pinus edulis*
Spruce, Hemlock	*Tsuga canadensis*

CITRUS AROMAS

Essential Oil	Latin name
Bergamot	Citrus bergamia
Grapefruit	*Citrus × paradisi*
Lemon	*Citrus limon*
Lime	*Citrus × aurantifolia*
Sweet Orange	*Citrus sinensis*
Mandarin	*Citrus reticulata*

Essential Oil	Latin name
Black Pepper	*Piper nigrum*
Cardamom	*Elettaria cardamomum*
Cinnamon Leaf	*Cinnamomum verum* (syn. *Cinnamomum zeylanicum)*
Clove Bud	*Syzygium aromaticum*
Ginger	*Zingiber officinale*
Turmeric	*Curcuma longa*

FLORAL AROMAS

Common Name	Latin name
Geranium	*Pelargonium × asperum*
Jasmine	*Jasminum grandiflorum* (or *Jasminum officinale)*
Lavender	*Lavandula angustifolia*
Neroli	*Citrus aurantium* var. *amara*
Petitgrain	*Citrus aurantium* var. *amara*
Rose	*Rosa × damascena* or *Rosa alba*
Ylang Ylang	*Cananga odorata*

RESIN AROMAS

Essential Oil	Latin name
Frankincense	*Boswellia sacra* (syn. *Boswellia carteri)*
Myrrh	*Commiphora myrrha*

THERAPEUTICS BY SYSTEM AFFINITY

SYSTEM AFFINITY	THERAPEUTICS
Circulatory (cardiovascular) system	**To support healthy circulation:** Black Pepper, Celery Seed, Juniper Berry, Lemon, Rosemary ct. cineole **Varicose veins,** to improve appearance of or prevent them from getting worse: Cypress, Lemon, Patchouli, Rose
Digestive system	**Relieve nausea:** Ginger, Peppermint **Relieve excess gas:** Anise, Cardamom, Cilantro, Coriander Seed, Sweet Fennel, Ginger, Peppermint **To support and enhance the digestive system (stimulating):** Anise, Black Pepper, Carrot Seed, Celery Seed, Sweet Fennel, Fingerroot, Ginger, Peppermint
Musculoskeletal system	**To relieve pain:** Roman Chamomile, Clary Sage, Clove Bud, Coriander Seed, Ginger, Laurel, Lemongrass, Sweet Marjoram, Peppermint, Plai, Rosemary ct. camphor, Vetiver, Wintergreen **To relieve muscle spasms:** Bergamot Mint, Roman Chamomile, Clary Sage, Coriander Seed, Lavender, Sweet Marjoram **To relieve muscular tension:** Basil ct. linalool, Bergamot Mint, Roman Chamomile, Clary Sage, Coriander Seed, Katafray, Lavender, Sweet Marjoram, Pinyon Pine, Hemlock Spruce, Vetiver To support recovery from sprains, strains, and repetitive injuries, herbal oils such as Arnica and St. John's wort can play a central role with essential oils.
Respiratory system	**Allergies:** to prevent or relieve allergies, use a personal inhaler: Blue Tansy, German Chamomile, Goldenrod **Decongesting and helpful for eliminating excess mucus in the nasal cavity:** Cardamom, Blue Gum Eucalyptus, Fingerroot, Laurel, Green Myrtle, Niaouli, Peppermint, Rosemary ct. cineole, Saro

$\rightarrow$

SYSTEM AFFINITY	THERAPEUTICS
Respiratory system (cont.)	**Immune Supportive Essential Oils:** Frankincense, Laurel, Niaouli, Hemlock Spruce, Lemon, Thyme ct. thymol
	Relieve spasmodic cough: Cardamom, Cypress, Laurel, Saro
	Help to clear congestion in lungs: Anise, Cardamom, Blue Gum Eucalyptus, Fingerroot, Inula, Laurel, Green Myrtle, Rosemary ct. cineole, Saro
Reproductive system	**For painful menstrual cramps or menstrual periods:** Clary Sage, Sweet Fennel, Lavender, Sweet Marjoram, Plai
	To uplift during challenging times, mood swings, or mild depression: Bergamot, Clary Sage, Neroli, Sweet Orange, Patchouli, Petitgrain, Mandarin, Rose, Ylang Ylang
	To increase sexual desire/aphrodisiacs: Cardamom, Cinnamon Leaf, Clary Sage, Ginger, Jasmine Absolute, Patchouli, Rose, Ylang Ylang
	To support hormonal balance: Clary Sage, Geranium, Lavender

THERAPEUTIC BENEFITS TO THE SKIN

ACTIVITY	ESSENTIAL OILS
Antimicrobial to support the skin in dealing with mild skin infections	Cistus, Lavender, Lemon, Melissa, Niaouli, Palmarosa, Thyme ct. linalool
Reduces inflammation of eczema, psoriasis, insect bites, rosacea, mild burns, sunburn, etc.	Calendula CO_2, Cape Chamomile, German Chamomile, Roman Chamomile, Copaiba, Frankincense, Lavender, Petitgrain, Blue Tansy, Yarrow
Relieves itchiness	Cape Chamomile, German chamomile, Lavender, Blue Tansy

$\rightarrow$

ACTIVITY	ESSENTIAL OILS
Astringent-like for excess oil, acne	Himalayan Cedarwood, Cypress, Neroli, Palmarosa, Patchouli, Rose
Cell regenerative as a preventative to aging and for skin rejuvenation	Calendula CO_2, Cistus, Frankincense, Lavender, Neroli, Palmarosa, Patchouli, Rose, Yarrow
Emollient to soften and soothe skin	Carrier oils, herbal oils, creams, lotions
Wound healing including poorly or slowly healing wounds	Calendula CO_2, Cistus, Frankincense, Lavender, Neroli, Palmarosa, Rose, Rosemary ct. verbenone, Yarrow
Nervine to reduce the impact of stress on the skin	Bergamot, Himalayan Cedarwood, Cape Chamomile, Roman Chamomile, German Chamomile, Frankincense, Lavender, Sweet Marjoram, Melissa, Neroli, Sweet Orange, Patchouli, Petitgrain, Rose, Mandarin, Vetiver, Yarrow, Ylang Ylang

EMOTIONS

In this emotion-based blending method, we are using the information contained in the plant part to send energetic message via its aroma. Also called Morphology, this method was developed by Jade Shutes early in her aromatherapy career and was first published in her *Blending Manual* in 1992. Other aromatherapy educators and books have since shared this approach to blending and selecting essential oils.

Blending by Morphology approaches the client and the essential oils based upon the unique message that each individual oil contains, based upon the part of the plant they are obtained from—seeds, roots, wood, resins, leaves or needles, flowers, or fruits. The chart below provides indications and examples of essential oils covered in this book for each category.

THERAPUTIC BENEFITS FOR EMOTIONS

PART OF PLANT	INDICATED FOR	ESSENTIAL OILS
Seeds	Inability to manifest, frustration, lack of communication between two people, inability to digest one's food and/or to gain nourishment, exhaustion, having difficulty conceiving ideas, boredom or inability to be in the present moment, imbalances of the second chakra or the solar plexus chakra, frigidity, hopelessness, cynicism, lack of self-esteem, frustration	Angelica Seed, Coriander Seed
Roots	Flightiness, instability, anxiety, feelings of being overwhelmed, scattered, sensitive constitution, nervousness, feelings of being disconnected to life, frazzled nerves, envy, compulsiveness, panic attacks, irritability, worry	Angelica Root, Ginger, Vetiver
Wood	Insecurity, lack of self-esteem, a need to go inward, self-reflection, need to conduct energy either upwards or downwards, weak constitution, envy	Himalayan Cedarwood
Resins	Post-traumatic stress, emotional wounds, anxiety, feelings of frustration, irritability, poor or lack of self-esteem, spiritual void or challenges, recovery from addictions or abuse, psychic wounding, lack of self-love and/or nourishment, impatience, tension, worry, despondency, bitterness, anger, anxiety	Copaiba, Frankincense, Myrrh

PART OF PLANT	INDICATED FOR	ESSENTIAL OILS
Leaves and Needles	Lack of confidence and/or self-esteem issues, shallow breathing, feelings of being hemmed in by life, contracted unable to expand, difficulty expressing emotions, stagnation, unable to shift or change/grow, lack of vitality, lack of courage, irritability, tension	Cypress, Blue Gum Eucalyptus, Balsam Fir, Laurel, Green Myrtle, Niaouli, Petitgrain, Peppermint, Pinyon Pine, Hemlock Spruce
Flowers	Anger, anxiety, burnout, lack of confidence, being critical of others, depression, despondency, lack of empathy, emptiness, frigidity, grief, grumpiness, guilt feelings, hopelessness, hostility, jealousy, Insecurity, instability, resentment, resignation, sadness, self-criticism (to bring back into body, inner awareness), self-esteem issues, shyness, stress, tension, inability to forgive	Roman Chamomile, German Chamomile, Clary Sage, Jasmine, Lavender, Neroli, Rose, Yarrow, Ylang Ylang
Fruits	Toxic thinking that turns in on the self, anger, self-criticism, cynicism, mild depression, despondency, frigidity, grief, grumpiness, guilt feelings, hopelessness, hostility, inability to forgive or let go, indecision (when decision is creating anxiety), insecurity, resentment, resignation, sadness, stress, tension	Bergamot, Grapefruit, Lemon, Mandarin, Sweet Orange

SYSTEM AFFINITY REVIEW

BODY SYSTEM	ESSENTIAL OILS
Circulatory	Black Pepper, Celery Seed, Cypress, Juniper Berry, Lemon, Rose, Rosemary ct. cineole
Reproductive	Clary Sage, Jasmine Absolute, Lavender, Mandarin, Sweet Marjoram, Neroli, Petitgrain, Plai, Rose
Digestive	Angelica Root, Bergamot, Black Pepper, Celery Seed, German Chamomile, Roman Chamomile, Cilantro, Coriander Seed, Fingerroot, Ginger, Grapefruit, Lemon, Mandarin, Sweet Orange, Peppermint, Thyme ct., thymol, Thyme ct. linalool
Musculoskeletal	Bergamot Mint, Black Pepper, Himalayan Cedarwood, Roman Chamomile, Clary Sage, Clove Bud, Coriander Seed, Ginger, Juniper Berry, Katafray, Laurel, Lavender, Lemongrass, Sweet Marjoram, Peppermint, Plai, Pinyon Pine, Rosemary ct. cineole , Rosemary ct. camphor, Hemlock, Spruce , Vetiver
Respiratory	Blue Tansy, Cypress, Eucalyptus Globulus, Fingerroot, Balsam Fir, Inula, Laurel, Sweet Marjoram, Green Myrtle, Niaouli, Peppermint, Pinyon Pine, Plai, Rosemary ct. cineole, Rosemary ct. camphor, Saro, Hemlock Spruce, Thyme ct. thymol
Skin	Calendula CO_2, Cape Chamomile, Himalayan Cedarwood, German Chamomile, Roman Chamomile, Cistus , Copaiba, Cypress, Frankincense, Lavender, Melissa, Neroli, Niaoul,i Palmarosa, Patchouli, Petitgrain, Rose, Rosemary ct. verbenone, Blue Tansy, Thyme ct. linalool, Yarrow

Endnotes

1. Shutes, J. (2000). Foundations of Aromatherapy certificate coursebook. New York Institute of Aromatic Studies.
2. Holmes, P. (2016). *Aromatica: A Clinical Guide to Essential Oil Therapeutics.* Volume 1: Principles and Profiles, Philadelphia, PA: Singing Dragon.
3. IBID
4. Tisserand, R. and Young, R. (2014) *Essential Oil Safety*, 2nd Edition. Milton, ON, CA: Churchill Livingstone Elsevier.
5. Mills, S. and Bone K. (2012). *Principles and Practice of Phytotherapy: Modern Herbal Medicine.* Milton, ON, CA: Churchill Livingstone Elsevier.
6. Mills, S. and Bone K. (2012). *Principles and Practice of Phytotherapy: Modern Herbal Medicine.* Milton, ON, CA: Churchill Livingstone Elsevier.
7. Schnaubelt, K. (2011). *The Healing Intelligence of Essential Oils: The Science of Advanced Aromatherapy.* Rochester, VT: Healing Arts Press.

Acknowledgments

To Jan Kusmirek, for inspiring me to think outside the box of traditional aromatherapy and to my son, Soren, for his love and support.
  –JS

I could not have written this book without the love and support from my husband, my parents, my mother-in-law, my sisters-in-law, my brother-in-law, my nephews, and my entire extended family. I also want to deeply thank all the students who passed through the doors of my school, The New York Institute of Aromatherapy, and the gifted team of teachers, Amy Anthony, Amandine Peter, and Elisabeth Vlasic, whose recipes are shared within the chapters of this book. A special thanks is also due to Celeste Knopf, who continues to make sure our work is accessible and shared. A huge shout out to Jill Alexander, our editor, who shepherded this book to manifest–along with the whole team at Fair Winds Press who made this possible. Baruch Hashem!

About the Authors

JADE SHUTES, B.A., Dipl. AT, Cert. Herbalist, has been practicing and studying forms of natural healing for nearly three decades. She was one of the vanguard of professionals who helped introduce aromatherapy to the US in the early 1990s. A prolific writer, Jade has influenced a generation of aromatherapy practitioners and home users with her balanced and progressive approach to the use of essential oils. She is the former President of National Association for Holistic Aromatherapy (NAHA). Her course Aromatic Medicine was a landmark course providing worldwide education on the internal use of essential oils.

An aromatherapy educator for over thirty years, Jade opened one of the first aromatherapy schools in United States. Jade spends much of her time in the Appalachia mountains of Virginia growing and distilling aromatic plants on her land, offering retreats, and expanding her relationship with the land and her community.

AMY GALPER, B.A., M.A., has been a certified aromatherapist since 2001, as well as a passionate advocate, entrepreneur, formulator, and consultant in clean beauty and wellness. She is the co-author of *Plant Powered Beauty* and endorsed by beauty industry visionary Bobbi Brown, Credo Beauty's Annie Jackson, Sophie Uliano, and Tata Harper. Amy is a member of Credo Beauty's Clean Beauty Council, celebrating, advocating and educating for Clean Beauty and Wellness, along with other influencers and thought leaders in the field.

She is a guest lecturer at New York University and has presented at Nova Southeastern University (NSU). She has been featured on Fox News, Thrive, Reuters, and has been quoted as an aromatherapy expert for countless print articles, television, podcasts, and online posts.

Contributors

AMY ANTHONY is a certified clinical aromatherapist, certified Aromatic Studies Method teacher, herbalist, gardener, and artisanal distiller with a private aromatherapy practice based in Manhattan. She is a graduate of the New York Institute of Aromatherapy where she earned her level 1 and level 2 aromatherapy certifications and is registered with the National Association for Holistic Aromatherapy. Read more of Amy's writing and about her practice at https://nycaroma.com.

AMANDINE PETER graduated from the New York Institute of Aromatic Studies, and eventually became a certified clinical aromatherapist and a certified Aromatic Studies Method teacher. In 2017, following her desire to harmonize aromatherapy with other healing modalities, she became a reiki master. She also teaches aromatherapy and herbalism classes at the New York Botanical Garden since 2018.

ELISABETH VLASIC, please call her Libby, is a certified aromatherapist and essential oil educator. She is a certified herbalist having attended Arbor Vitae School of Traditional Herbalism in New York City. A dedicated forever student of the plant-world, Libby was honored to be a senior teacher at the New York Institute of Aromatic Studies for many years.

Index

Roman Chamomile (*Chamaemelum nobile* syn. *Anthemis nobilis,* Asteraceae), 34

roots, 150

Rose *(Rosa × damascena),* 8, 113

Rose geranium *(Pelargonium graveolens* var. *roseum),* 112

rosehip seed oil, 106

rosemary, 14

Rosemary (*Rosmarinus officinalis,* Lamiaceae), 72–73

    containing camphor, 72–73

    containing, verbenone, 73

S

safety, 20

sage, 14

salt scrubs, 123–24

salves, 121–22

Saro (*Cinnamosma fragrans,* Canellaceae), 74

sea buckthorn oil, 106

seeds, 150

sensitization, 15–6

sesame oil, 107

Shea butter *(Vitellaria paradoxa* (syn. *Butyrospermum parkii)),* 109

skin, therapeutic benefits to, 148–49

smelling salts, 135–36

spicy aromas, 146

St. John's wort *(Hypericum perforatum),* 108

steam inhalation, 136–37

strong essential oils, 13–14

sunflower oil, 107

Sweet Marjoram (*Origanum majorana,* Lamiaceae), 80

Sweet Orange (*Citrus sinensis,* Rutaceae), 39

synergy, formulating, 142–43

system affinities, 20–21

    circulatory (cardiovascular system), 147

    digestive system, 147

    musculoskeletal system, 147

    reproductive system, 148

    respiratory system, 147–48

T

tamanu oil, 107

therapeutic applications, 21–22. *See also* various essential oils

Thyme (*Thymus vulgaris,* Lamiaceae), 98–99

V

Valerian (*Valeriana officinalis,* Caprifoliaceae), 29

Vetiver (*Chrysopogon zizanioides* syn. *Vetiveria zizanioides,* Poaceae), 54

W

waxes, 110–11

Witch hazel *(Hamamelis virginiana),* 113

wood, 150

wormwood, 14

Y

Yarrow (*Achillea millefolium,* Asteraceae), 95

Ylang Ylang (*Cananga odorata,* Annonaceae), 59

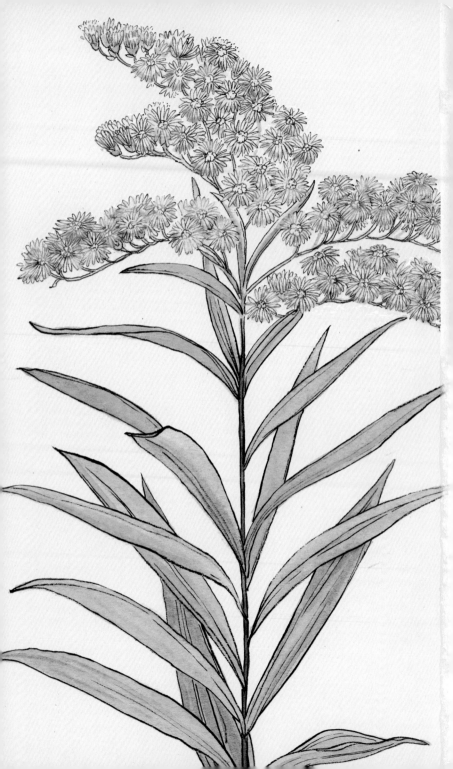